Tables

Figures

Boxes

Summary

Ohe of lawmakers' highest health-related priorities is adding a prescription drug benefit to Medicare. Although that program gives older Americans broad insurance coverage for many health needs, it provides only limited coverage of drugs not dispensed during a hospital stay. That gap in coverage has become increasingly significant as prescription drugs have assumed greater importance in the treatment of disease and as spending for outpatient prescription drugs has soared.

Designing a Medicare drug benefit is a complex task, however. The competing goals for such a benefit mean that policymakers must make trade-offs (such as between broad coverage or widespread enrollment and cost). They must consider many different design elements and how those elements might interact. And they must try to avoid various problems that arise in creating such a benefit. Ultimately, the choices that designers make will affect not only the cost of the benefit but a host of other factors, such as demand for and prices of prescription drugs, spending by other federal and state programs, and how various parts of the market for health insurance operate.

The Congressional Budget Office (CBO) has had to wrestle with those issues in recent years to produce cost estimates of the various Medicare drug proposals debated in the Congress. This study summarizes the main design choices facing policymakers and explores the implications of those choices for cost and coverage. To illustrate the effect of those choices on cost, it also discusses CBO's cost estimates for four proposals that represent a broad array of designs for a Medicare drug benefit.

For the sake of simplicity, this study focuses on a stand-alone drug benefit—one that would be a freestanding addition to Medicare rather than part of a broad effort to restructure the program. Broad reform proposals raise important policy issues but ones that are beyond the scope of this analysis.

Higher Drug Costs and Declining Coverage Are Spurring Calls for a Medicare Drug Benefit

Spending for prescription drugs is the fastest growing segment of U.S. health care costs. And Medicare beneficiaries (people who are 65 or older or disabled) account for a disproportionate share of that spending: about 40 percent, although they make up less than 15 percent of the U.S. population. CBO expects Medicare beneficiaries' drug costs to rise rapidly over the next decade (even without adding a drug benefit to Medicare)—at a per-beneficiary rate of 10.1 percent a year, on average. That rate is much faster than the projected growth of spending for current Medicare benefits, and more than twice as fast as the expected per capita growth of the U.S. economy.

This year, Medicare beneficiaries will use a total of almost $87 billion in outpatient prescription drugs. That figure is projected to rise to more than $128 billion by 2005, the earliest year that Medicare could probably begin implementing a drug benefit that was enacted in 2002.

Although most Medicare beneficiaries use some prescription drugs, that spending is concentrated among a relatively small part of the Medicare population: people with chronic conditions requiring long-term drug therapy. Only 17 percent of Medicare beneficiaries will spend more than $5,000 on prescription drugs in 2005, CBO estimates, but their combined spending will make up nearly 54 percent of total drug expenditures by Medicare beneficiaries that year.

Roughly one-quarter of Medicare beneficiaries have no prescription drug coverage (as of 1999, the most recent year for which data are available). Thus, they must pay all of their drug costs out of pocket. The other three-quarters obtain drug coverage as part of a plan that supplements Medicare's benefits. But those supplemental plans differ greatly in the extent of coverage they provide. And recent trends suggest that the availability and comprehensiveness of supplemental drug coverage may be declining. Many employment-based health plans for retirees have been scaling back drug benefits in the face of rising costs. The same is true of managed care plans that participate in the Medicare+Choice program, some of which offer drug coverage as an additional benefit.

Medicare beneficiaries who have drug coverage had an average of about 32 prescriptions filled in 1999. The one-quarter of Medicare beneficiaries without drug coverage used fewer prescription drugs that year—but still had an average of 25 prescriptions filled. Medicare beneficiaries who lack drug coverage tend to be people in the low to middle part of the income distribution. People with higher income are more likely to have employment-based plans or individually purchased medigap policies (which charge high premiums for drug coverage). People with the lowest income qualify for drug benefits from Medicaid or from state-sponsored pharmaceutical assistance programs.

Proposals that would target Medicare drug coverage toward low- to middle-income beneficiaries who are not eligible for Medicaid would concentrate new federal spending on those least likely to have drug coverage now. Broad-based proposals, by contrast, would tend to replace coverage that three-fourths of beneficiaries now get from private and nonfederal sources with Medicare-funded coverage. CBO expects that broad-based proposals for a Medicare drug benefit would redistribute some drug financing from employers and states to Medicare.

Design Choices for a Medicare Drug Benefit Must Balance Competing Objectives

Policymakers cite various goals for a Medicare prescription drug benefit, some of which may be incompatible. Those goals include making sure that all Medicare beneficiaries have access to drug coverage, offering coverage that is relatively comprehensive and that reimburses some share of costs for most enrollees, providing insurance protection for elderly people who have the highest drug spending, ensuring that enrollees' premiums are affordable, and limiting the cost to the federal government.

A Medicare drug benefit could require substantial federal spending, especially if the government subsidized a large share of the costs for many enrollees. Medicare beneficiaries are expected to spend an average of nearly $2,500 apiece on outpatient prescription drugs next year, and access to better drug coverage would undoubtedly stimulate further spending. However, policymakers could exacerbate or alleviate the federal cost burden through their decisions about the design of the benefit.

How Comprehensive Will the Benefit Be?

The most important factor determining the cost of a Medicare drug benefit is the scope and structure of its coverage. Choices about coverage include:

■ The deductible amount—whether coverage begins with an enrollee's first dollar of drug spending in a given year or after the deductible amount is reached;

■ Cost-sharing rates—what part of the cost of a prescription is the responsibility of the enrollee;

■ The benefit cap—the level of spending beyond which the enrollee must pay the full cost of each prescription; and

■ The catastrophic stop-loss amount—the level of spending beyond which the enrollee pays little or nothing for prescriptions.

The possible variations on those choices are endless. Some combinations could produce Medicare drug benefits unlike anything available in the private sector today. (For example, many of the recent Medicare proposals envision a hole in coverage: a spending level between the benefit cap and the stop-loss amount at which enrollees would have no drug coverage. Employment-based drug plans almost never include such holes.)

The benefit structure would affect the cost of the Medicare drug program not only directly but also indirectly, through the out-of-pocket expenses it would require of enrollees. For instance, benefits with low cost-sharing rates would encourage those enrollees who were newly shielded from paying the full cost of a prescription to use more—and more expensive—drugs.

Who Will Be Eligible to Enroll?

Choices about eligibility include whether the prescription drug benefit would be available to all Medicare beneficiaries or only to some (such as those with low income, few assets, or no current drug coverage). Another key decision is whether to make enrollment in the drug benefit voluntary and, if so, with what restrictions. If the benefit was voluntary and did not limit when and how often eligible people could enroll, Medicare beneficiaries would tend to sign up (and pay premiums) only when they expected to incur high drug costs; they would opt out again when they foresaw little need for prescription drugs. As a result, the cost of the program per participant would be higher than if people had to enroll and pay premiums for a longer period of time.

How Much Will the Government Subsidize?

To what extent will the government pay enrollees' costs for premiums or prescriptions? And will those subsidies vary with enrollees' income? Those design choices affect not only federal spending but also spending by state and local governments, which help pay the drug costs of some

low-income elderly people through Medicaid and other programs. In addition, the level of subsidy offered to Medicare beneficiaries would have an important effect on people's willingness to enroll in the drug program.

How Will the Benefit Be Administered?

Almost all of the recent proposals for a Medicare drug benefit envision using organizations such as pharmacy benefit managers (PBMs) to administer the benefit—an approach that is common in the private sector. Critical choices, however, are the number of such organizations that would serve a region, the restrictions they would be subject to, the basis on which they could compete for enrollees, and whether they would assume any insurance risk (that is, be liable for any costs that were not fully covered by enrollees' premiums or federal reimbursements).

In examining prescription drug proposals, CBO has concluded that certain administrative features offer the greatest opportunity to control federal costs and total spending on outpatient prescription drugs. Those features are allowing benefit managers to employ the full array of cost-management tools now available to private-sector drug plans, forcing benefit managers to compete among themselves for enrollees' business, and making managers assume financial risk for delivering benefits.

Benefit Designs Must Address Multiple Problems

In making the design choices described above, policymakers need to consider several problems inherent in creating a Medicare drug benefit. Those problems include the possibility that the coverage will mainly attract people with the highest drug costs, the need to limit costs to the government and to enrollees, the ability and willingness of private entities (such as health insurers and PBMs) to administer the drug benefit, and the possible impact of the benefit on other parts of the Medicare program.

Adverse Selection

A stand-alone prescription drug benefit could be especially prone to the insurance-market phenomenon known as adverse selection, in which people who expect to have higher-than-average costs disproportionately enroll in an insurance plan. Adverse selection can occur when plans (or potential enrollees) make decisions based on the desire to avoid attracting (or being grouped with) enrollees who are likely to have expensive claims. For example, health insurers can design their coverage or market their plans in ways that will be especially attractive to relatively healthy people. And potential enrollees who would rather not be in an insurance pool with people who are likely to have high costs—because that would imply higher premiums than would otherwise be the case—may opt out of insurance altogether.

Adverse selection is a problem because it undermines the purpose of insurance, which is to spread financial risks among a wide pool of people. Adverse selection raises the cost of insurance for people who do enroll. And it makes people who are discouraged from enrolling worse off by not receiving the benefits of insurance. (Even people who expect to have low medical costs could benefit from insuring against the possibility that they develop a serious illness.) The outcome of adverse selection can be a pattern of high premiums and low enrollment, resulting in much less coverage than would exist otherwise.

Two kinds of adverse selection could affect the operation of a Medicare drug benefit: adverse selection into the drug program as a whole; and, if multiple plans are allowed to administer the drug benefit in the same region and bear financial risk for the cost of the benefit, adverse selection among those plans.

Adverse Selection into the Drug Program. If relatively healthy Medicare beneficiaries (such as those with no chronic conditions) tended to opt out of Medicare drug coverage, costs and premiums would be higher for people who did enroll than they would be if the benefit covered a representative mix of Medicare beneficiaries. Paradoxically, although adverse selection into the drug program would raise costs per enrollee, it would most likely reduce the total cost of the drug benefit, because the number of participants would be so much smaller. Such a situation could become unstable, however, with premiums continuing to grow and enrollment continuing to drop.

The main way to prevent adverse selection into the drug program would be to encourage as many people as possible to enroll. The government could do that through a number of approaches:

- *Requiring One-Time Enrollment.* A "choose it or lose it" policy would boost enrollment because even healthy Medicare beneficiaries might be worried enough about developing an expensive medical condition someday that they would enroll in the drug benefit if they had only one chance to do so.

- *Subsidizing the Program to a Large Extent.* Broad federal subsidies would mean that even fairly healthy people would be likely to get more in benefits than they paid in premiums.

- *Risk-Rating Premiums.* Adjusting the premiums that enrollees would pay according to their risk of high drug spending would encourage healthier people to enroll because their costs would be lower.

- *Making the Drug Benefit a Mandatory Part of Medicare's Part B.* If drug coverage was incorporated into Medicare's Supplementary Medical Insurance benefits, even people who expected to have low drug costs would be inclined to enroll in order to insure against the general medical expenses they might face.

Adverse Selection Among Drug Plans. When a prescription drug program allows competing plans to operate and requires them to assume financial risk for the benefits they pay out, difficulties related to interplan adverse selection can result. That type of adverse selection occurs when certain plans attract beneficiaries with high expected costs because their services or coverage are more generous than are those of other plans. Drug plans would probably react to the possibility of adverse selection by trying to avoid enrolling people who are apt to have high drug costs. For example, they might advertise their plans at golf clubs but not at nursing homes. Or they might cap benefits below the spending levels likely to be reached by seniors with chronic health conditions, or they might require substantial cost sharing.

The government could employ various policy tools to minimize interplan adverse selection: it could require plans to offer standardized benefits or could create standardized marketing materials for all Medicare drug plans, or it could compensate plans for their differential costs through reinsurance or risk adjustment. In addition, as noted above, the government could allow drug plans to charge risk-rated premiums.

Strategies that would reduce adverse selection, however, could create other problems. Perhaps the most significant is that if plans were shielded from the full burden of high spending, they would have less incentive to control costs. Thus, reducing the risks associated with interplan adverse selection must be weighed against plans' incentive to control costs.

Cost Containment

Medicare spending is expected to soar over the next three decades as the large baby-boom generation becomes eligible for the program. Adding subsidized drug coverage to Medicare would significantly increase the federal government's financial commitment, particularly since Medicare beneficiaries' drug spending is projected to grow at double-digit rates each year even without a drug benefit. Thus, controlling costs is a key problem in designing such a benefit.

The extent of the cost containment challenge depends on the level of coverage provided. A more extensive benefit would shift more of the burden of paying for drugs from consumers to drug plans. In addition, by reducing out-of-pocket costs to enrollees, a Medicare drug benefit would stimulate demand for prescription drugs. The more generous the coverage (the lower the deductible, the required cost sharing, and the catastrophic stop-loss amount), the greater would be the stimulus to demand—and the greater the burden on cost management to limit that growth in demand.

Active cost management by the entities administering the Medicare drug benefit could encourage the use of fewer or less-expensive drugs. The degree to which PBMs could effectively control Medicare drug costs would depend on their being allowed and encouraged to aggressively use the various tools at their disposal. Those tools include formularies (lists of drugs that a health plan will cover) and related approaches that steer demand to preferred drugs, networks of pharmacies, disease-management programs, and efforts to educate patients and physicians. All of those tools, to one degree or another, work by influencing physicians' or consumers' choices about what drug to prescribe or where to fill a prescription.

In addition, requiring benefit managers to assume some insurance risk for the benefits they pay out and allowing multiple entities to compete for enrollees on the basis of premiums and reimbursements would give managers a greater incentive to hold down spending. However, the savings from those features would be partly offset by two kinds of additional costs:

■ *The Insurance-Risk Premium.* Riskier enterprises require higher dollar returns to operate than less risky ones do, because unless investors are compensated for bearing the extra risk, investment in those enterprises will dry up. A design that made PBMs or other benefit administrators bear insurance risk would impose a higher cost on those entities than would a design that left insurance risk in the hands of the government. That added cost is referred to as the insurance-risk premium.

■ *Plans' Marketing Costs.* Competition would introduce additional expenses associated with marketing to and enrolling Medicare beneficiaries, which would not arise if a single plan administered the drug benefit in each region. Competing plans would have to provide specific information about their plans to beneficiaries. If plans were also responsible for enrolling people and collecting their premiums, the cost of carrying out those administrative functions would be higher than under a single-plan system.

Ways exist to keep the insurance-risk premium and marketing costs in check without losing most of the savings from a competitive system with active benefit management. One approach would be to limit insurance risk by providing reinsurance to plans for very high cost enrollees. Under one type of reinsurance mechanism, a drug plan would receive government funds on the basis of the claims incurred by each of its enrollees. If an enrollee's claims in a year reached a specific level, the government would pay the plan a certain fraction of the enrollee's additional claims costs. That fraction would increase as the enrollee's claims grew. With such a mechanism, plans would still have an incentive to actively manage the drug benefit, but they would be protected from uncontrollably high-cost enrollees.

The extra marketing and administrative costs associated with competition could also be reduced (though not eliminated) by standardizing the information given to Medicare beneficiaries, by having the government perform the functions of enrolling beneficiaries and collecting premiums, and by facilitating efficient marketing to prospective enrollees.

Even the most effective benefit management, however, would not keep the prices of some drugs from rising under a Medicare drug benefit. By raising the limit on consumers' willingness or ability to pay for covered drugs, a generous drug benefit would make newly insured patients more tolerant of high prices. With such a benefit, if a manufacturer developed a unique drug whose target population consisted mainly of Medicare beneficiaries, it could raise the drug's price (or, if the drug was new, enter the market with a high launch price). Preventing very high prices for such drugs would be difficult apart from imposing direct price controls or threatening to deny or delay coverage of the drug—actions that could increase uncertainty about the market for new drugs and thus discourage investment in pharmaceutical research and development.

Fortunately, most drugs are not unique but instead face competition from close substitutes. For such drugs, the most likely effect of a Medicare drug benefit would be only moderate price increases, and then only for drugs with patent protection or exclusive marketing rights. Nevertheless, the possibility that manufacturers of patent-protected drugs could raise prices underscores the impor-

tance of giving benefit managers both the incentive and the authority to use cost-management tools.

Administrative Feasibility

Some proposals would require the private organizations charged with administering the Medicare drug benefit not only to play the roles that PBMs do in the private sector but also to compete for enrollees, bear insurance risk, and cope with federal (and possibly state) regulation. An important area of uncertainty is whether private entities would be willing or able to participate in the Medicare drug program under those conditions. If they were not, the program would take longer and cost more to implement nationwide.

Private organizations could face at least three barriers to participation. First, in order to compete as risk-bearing entities, most PBMs would probably have to form partnerships with insurance companies and seek state licenses. Alternatively, PBMs could offer their traditional benefit-management services to insurance companies that would provide the Medicare drug benefit. In either case, new functional roles and relationships would need to be developed before private entities could bid to offer Medicare drug plans. Second, plans might be reluctant to enter the market early because of uncertainty about how competition among plans would work itself out. Especially in the early years of the program, plans might be unable to gauge their risk of interplan adverse selection or know how effective their strategies to cope with such risk would be. And third, plans would face regulatory hurdles unless the states' role in licensing and regulating participating drug plans was clarified at the outset.

It is possible that only one plan or even no plans would participate in the drug program in some areas. Without multiple plans in a region, the full benefits of competition would not be realized. If that happened, the government might have to provide its own public plan as a fallback in those areas (or offer extra financial incentives for private plans to operate there) to ensure a competitive program nationwide. Fallback plans would be very vulnerable to interplan adverse selection in any region where there was also a risk-bearing plan. If the fallback plan was less aggressive than other plans in managing costs, the government could end up paying more, on average, in areas requiring such direct intervention.

Impact on Other Parts of Medicare

Adding a stand-alone prescription drug benefit to Medicare would have ripple effects on the rest of the program. For some seniors, greater access to outpatient prescription drugs would improve their health, reducing their use of hospitals and other services that Medicare now covers. For other seniors, however, use of health care could increase. For example, using a greater number of drugs raises the probability of adverse events—such as harmful drug interactions or side effects—which could lead to new or longer visits to hospitals, emergency rooms, and other health care providers. Little good evidence exists from which to determine the net effect of drug coverage on other Medicare services; but overall, costs for other Medicare services would probably not change significantly.

One part of Medicare that would most likely be affected by the availability of a drug benefit is the Medicare+ Choice (M+C) program. Those effects would go in conflicting directions, however. On the one hand, the managed care plans that take part in the M+C program have historically attracted beneficiaries by offering benefits beyond the basic Medicare package—the most desirable of which is prescription drug coverage. If drug coverage was available to beneficiaries of regular fee-for-service Medicare, M+C plans would lose one of their principal competitive advantages.

On the other hand, under a Medicare drug benefit, M+C plans that offered drug coverage would be paid for the value of that coverage rather than having to finance it from their savings on administration or benefits. The rising cost of prescription drugs and the lack of Medicare payment for drug coverage (combined with 1997 changes in payment rates) are reasons that M+C plans have cited

for dropping out of Medicare in recent years. Higher payments, to cover the cost of a prescription drug benefit, could help stabilize those plans' participation.

Cost Estimates for Medicare Drug Proposals Reflect the Choices Made by Policymakers

In recent years, policymakers have offered a host of proposals for a Medicare prescription drug benefit. The types of design choices described above have a significant effect on those proposals' costs. Four Medicare drug proposals introduced during the 106th Congress (1999 to 2000) are particularly good examples of the broad spectrum of benefit designs being considered and the various ways in which a Medicare drug benefit could be administered. Each year, when CBO updates its 10-year projections of drug spending by or for Medicare beneficiaries, it also updates its estimates for those proposals as a way to evaluate its estimating methods and key assumptions. Those proposals are the benefit described in the Clinton Administration's June 2000 *Mid-Session Review;* the Robb amendment (introduced by Senator Charles Robb as amendment 3598 to H.R. 4577); H.R. 4680 (introduced by Representative William Thomas), which passed the House of Representatives in October 2000; and Breaux-Frist II (S. 2807, introduced by Senator John Breaux).

The original versions of those four proposals would have introduced a Medicare drug benefit in 2002 or 2003. In updating its estimates, CBO used the same dollar amounts included in the original proposals but assumed that the new Medicare drug program would begin in 2005. For example, if a proposal called for a $250 deductible and a stop-loss amount of $5,000 in out-of-pocket spending, CBO used those dollar values for 2005. (After that, it indexed them for projected changes in per capita drug spending through 2012, the end of the current 10-year budget window.) Keeping the same nominal values for the benefit's initial deductible and stop-loss amount while drug spending is growing tends to make the proposals more generous than when they were introduced. However, policymakers have been reluctant to propose a new Medicare drug benefit with higher deductibles and catastrophic stop-loss limits.

The Design of the Four Proposals

All four proposals would offer drug coverage on a voluntary basis as a new Part D of Medicare, but they would give beneficiaries only a one-time opportunity to enroll without penalty. (If beneficiaries delayed enrollment, they would pay a penalty related to their expected benefit costs when they signed up.) Without that provision, CBO would assume much lower rates of enrollment and much higher costs per enrollee for each proposal, because people would tend to postpone signing up for the benefit until their drug spending became relatively high.

The Clinton Administration's Plan. The proposal included in the Clinton Administration's 2000 *Mid-Session Review* called for a Medicare drug benefit that would have no deductible and would pay 50 percent of an enrollee's drug spending up to a limit of $1,000 in 2005 (*see Summary Table 1*). Once a participant incurred $4,000 in out-of-pocket costs during the year, Medicare would cover 100 percent of further drug spending. Under the proposal, plans would have the flexibility to vary their enrollees' coinsurance rates if they could demonstrate that the lower cost sharing would not raise costs for the Medicare program; that is, more-generous benefits would be offset by more-effective cost management.

The Secretary of Health and Human Services (HHS) would set a uniform national premium for the drug benefit. Enrollees with income of up to 150 percent of the federal poverty level would receive assistance in paying their premiums; those with income of up to 135 percent of the poverty level would also get help in paying their cost-sharing amounts. In addition, Medicare would offer a subsidy to employment-based health plans to encourage them to remain the primary payer for their retirees' drug coverage. (That subsidy would equal 67 percent of the amount that Medicare would have paid if a plan's retirees had enrolled in the Part D benefit.)

With those provisions, the general federal subsidy for all enrollees would equal 50 percent of "premium costs" (the total value of the benefits paid out plus the cost of administering the drug program) below the stop-loss limit. That subsidy would be 100 percent above the limit.

Under the Clinton Administration's proposal, PBMs or other entities would compete to be the sole Medicare drug plan in each geographic area for a specified period of time. PBMs would not bear insurance risk for their enrollees' drug spending, and they would face restrictions on the cost-management approaches they could use. For example, they would have to set dispensing fees high enough to ensure participation by most retail pharmacies. In addition, enrollees would be guaranteed access to any drug that the prescribing physician certified as medically necessary.

The Robb Amendment. Unlike the other proposals examined in this study, the Robb amendment would not cap an enrollee's benefits. Under that amendment, enrollees would pay a $250 deductible and graduated coinsurance rates—50 percent until their annual out-of-pocket drug spending reached $3,500, then 25 percent until their out-of-pocket spending reached $4,000. After that, Medicare would cover all of their additional drug spending. The entities selected to administer the benefit would be allowed to waive the deductible for generic drugs and to lower beneficiaries' coinsurance rates if they could show that the lower cost sharing would be offset by effective cost management.

Like the Clinton Administration's plan, the Robb amendment would have the Secretary of HHS set a uniform nationwide premium. The proposal would also provide low-income subsidies to cover premiums and cost sharing for enrollees with income of up to 135 percent of the poverty level and premium assistance for people with income of up to 150 percent of the poverty level. The Robb amendment would offer the same subsidy as the Clinton proposal to employment-based health plans if they remained the primary source of drug coverage for their retirees. The general subsidy for all enrollees would equal 50 percent of premium costs.

Unlike the Clinton Administration's proposal, however, the Robb amendment envisions a competitive system,

Summary Table 1.

Provisions of Four Prescription Drug Proposals for Medicare

	Clinton Mid-Session Review Plan	Robb Amendment	H.R. 4680	Breaux-Frist II
Benefit Amounts (Dollars)[a]				
Deductible	None	250	250	250
Benefit cap	1,000	None	1,050	1,050
Stop-loss amount	4,000	4,000	6,000	6,000
Benefit Administrator	SSA	SSA	Plans	SSA
Subsidies for Employment-Based Health Plans	Yes	Yes	No[b]	No[b]
Number of Plans in Each Region	One	At least two	At least two	At least two
Plans Bear Insurance Risk	No	No	Yes	Yes
Federal Subsidy for All Enrollees[c]	50% subsidy of premium costs below stop-loss amount; 100% above	50% subsidy of premium costs	No subsidy of premium costs; graduated reinsurance rate, averaging 35%[d]	25% subsidy of premium costs below stop-loss amount; 80% reinsurance above

Source: Congressional Budget Office.

Note: SSA = Social Security Administration.

a. The amounts that would apply in the Medicare drug benefit's first year of operation, which is assumed to be calendar year 2005.

b. Employment-based health plans for retirees could participate as entities that provide a Medicare drug plan, with the same federal subsidy as other plans. However, no attempt was made to estimate what share of total enrollment in the drug benefit they would account for.

c. "Premium costs" refers to the total value of the benefits paid out plus the cost of administering the drug program.

d. Today, the enrollee spending levels specified in H.R. 4680 at which federal reinsurance would be paid would lead to a federal subsidy of more than 35 percent. However, the legislative language caps that subsidy at 35 percent. Thus, the spending levels at which the federal government paid reinsurance would need to be raised.

with at least two entities (selected through competitive bidding) administering the drug benefit in each region. Those entities would not bear insurance risk for their enrollees' drug spending. They would also have fewer explicit restrictions on the tools they could employ to control drug spending than under the Clinton plan. For example, PBMs could use restrictive formularies, subject to rules set by a national committee. However, they would have to provide any drug approved for marketing in the United States if it was medically necessary for a patient (as established through procedures set by the PBM).

H.R. 4680. This proposal, which the House of Representatives passed in October 2000 but the Senate did not

consider, also envisioned a drug benefit with a $250 deductible. Medicare would pay 50 percent of participants' drug costs, up to a cap of $1,050 in the first year of the benefit. Once enrollees incurred out-of-pocket costs of $6,000 or more during the year, Medicare would cover 100 percent of their drug spending. H.R. 4680 would allow participating plans to offer actuarially equivalent versions of the standard benefit—subject to certain limits.

Multiple plans would compete for enrollees in each region on the basis of premiums, access to drugs, and quality of services (once they were approved by the agency administering the program through a process of negotiation). Unlike the two proposals discussed above, H.R. 4680 would require those plans to assume significant insurance risk. It would also allow them to use a broad array of tools to control their enrollees' drug spending.

The federal government would ensure that at least two plans were available in each area, one of which could be a Medicare+Choice plan offering drug coverage. Employment-based health plans for retirees would also be eligible to participate directly as entities themselves. In any area not served by at least two plans, Medicare would have authority to provide financial incentives (such as a partial underwriting of risk) to encourage plans to operate in that region.

Rather than having one nationwide premium set by Medicare, H.R. 4680 would allow entities to set their own premiums. As a result, premiums would vary geographically and among plans. Low-income subsidies would cover premiums and cost-sharing expenses for enrollees with income of up to 135 percent of the poverty level (except that those enrollees would be responsible for covering any spending in the hole between the benefit cap and the stop-loss amount). Enrollees with income of up to 150 percent of the poverty level would be eligible for assistance with their premiums.

Unlike in the other proposals, the federal government would not provide an across-the-board subsidy of each plan's premium. Instead, it would make reinsurance payments to plans for the spending of very high cost enrollees. In total, those payments would amount to 35 percent of the cost of benefits paid out under the drug program.

Breaux-Frist II. This proposal has the exact same benefit structure as H.R. 4680 and a similar subsidy for low-income enrollees. However, its provisions for the general federal subsidy for all enrollees differ. Whereas H.R. 4680 would provide all of that subsidy through individual reinsurance payments for high-cost enrollees, Breaux-Frist II would subsidize 25 percent of premium costs below the $6,000 catastrophic stop-loss limit and then cover 80 percent of benefits above that limit through individual reinsurance.

Multiple risk-bearing plans would offer the benefit in each region, and premiums could vary geographically and among plans. In addition, PBMs would have the same incentives and authority to manage costs under this proposal that they would have under H.R. 4680. However, unlike in H.R. 4680, the Social Security Administration would administer enrollment and collect premiums. As a result, plans' marketing and enrollment costs would be lower under this proposal than under H.R. 4680.

Summary Table 2.

Federal Costs of Four Prescription Drug Proposals, 2005-2012

(By fiscal year, in billions of dollars)

	Clinton Mid-Session Review Plan	Robb Amendment	H.R. 4680	Breaux-Frist II
Federal Mandatory Spending on Prescription Drug Benefits for Medicare Beneficiaries				
Medicare	507	342	120	178
Other federal programs[a]	-145	-142	-84	-78
Low-income subsidy	128	148	141	123
Other Mandatory Spending	22	27	18	10
Total	**512**	**374**	**195**	**233**

Source: Congressional Budget Office.

Note: These numbers exclude a small amount of appropriated funds for federal administrative costs.

a. Principally Medicaid, the Federal Employees Health Benefits program, and the military's Tricare for Life program. Negative numbers indicate savings.

Range of Cost Estimates for the Four Proposals

To estimate the costs of a proposed Medicare drug benefit, CBO uses a model that simulates how that benefit would affect the spending of a representative sample of Medicare beneficiaries. The model contains detailed information about Medicare beneficiaries' spending for prescription drugs and other health services, their supplemental insurance coverage, their health status, and their income. CBO's cost estimates result from running the model using a proposal's total design specifications; because the various design elements affect one another, the impact of specific design choices on costs cannot be quantified independently.

Among the four proposed drug benefits examined here, CBO estimates that the Clinton Administration's would have the highest costs to the federal government: a total of $512 billion between 2005 and 2012 (*see Summary Table 2*). That total reflects the federal costs of the new Medicare benefit, including subsidies for low-income enrollees, partly offset by federal savings in other programs, such as Medicaid, the Federal Employees Health Benefits program, and the military's Tricare for Life program. The Robb amendment would rank second in federal costs, at $374 billion over the same eight-year period. Breaux-Frist II and H.R. 4680 would cost $233 billion and $195 billion, respectively, during the 2005-2012 period. Although those two proposals have identical benefit structures, they differ in terms of the share of total costs subsidized by the federal government. As a result, their levels of enrollment would differ as well as their federal costs.

The federal costs of a particular drug benefit depend largely on the extent to which it subsidizes total drug spending by or for Medicare beneficiaries. Thus, the Robb and Clinton plans—which would pay 21 percent and 29 percent, respectively, of Medicare beneficiaries' total drug costs—would have the highest costs to Medicare. H.R. 4680 and Breaux-Frist II—which would pay for 12 percent to 15 percent of total drug spending by or for Medicare beneficiaries—would have lower costs to the Medicare program.

Introduction

Medicare offers broad insurance protection for many health needs of the nation's elderly. However, it provides very limited coverage for the costs of outpatient prescription drugs (those not dispensed during a hospital stay). That gap in coverage has become increasingly significant over the past three decades for a number of reasons. Prescription drugs have assumed growing importance in the treatment of disease, especially as new, more effective—and more costly—drugs have become available to treat chronic diseases prevalent in older people. Partly as a result, spending for outpatient prescription drugs has soared.

Despite Medicare's limited drug coverage, most beneficiaries have not faced the full effects of that rapid rise in spending. The reason is that roughly three-quarters of Medicare beneficiaries have insurance coverage for outpatient prescription drugs through other sources. Those sources include private insurance plans—such as employment-based plans for retirees and medigap plans that are specifically designed to supplement Medicare—as well as public programs, such as Medicaid. Some managed care plans in the Medicare+Choice program also offer drug coverage as an extra benefit, usually for an additional premium. In general, the Medicare beneficiaries who lack supplemental drug coverage or who have only limited coverage are people in the low to middle part of the income scale.

Policymakers have shown widespread interest in providing a comprehensive drug benefit through the Medicare program. They cite various goals for such a benefit, some of which may be mutually incompatible:

■ Ensuring that all Medicare beneficiaries have access to drug coverage,

■ Offering coverage that is relatively comprehensive and that reimburses some costs for most enrollees,

■ Providing insurance protection for elderly people with the highest drug spending,

■ Ensuring that premiums are affordable, and

■ Limiting the cost to the federal government.

The extent to which particular policy goals are met will depend largely on how the Medicare drug benefit is designed. Even seemingly minor differences in specific design features can have a big impact on the drug program's cost to the federal government, its impact on total spending for prescription drugs, and the level of insurance protection it affords enrollees. Moreover, different design features could have complex interactions. A clearer understanding of those differences and interactions would permit policymakers to better balance the trade-offs inherent in a Medicare prescription drug benefit, such as the trade-off between higher costs and greater insurance coverage.

The Congressional Budget Office (CBO) has grappled with many of those issues in estimating the costs of Medicare drug programs proposed during the past three sessions of Congress. This study summarizes the key design choices facing policymakers and explores the implications of those choices for cost and coverage. It also discusses CBO's cost estimates for four Medicare drug proposals first introduced in 1999 or 2000 during the 106th Congress. Those proposals are the one in the Clinton Administration's June 2000 *Mid-Session Review;* the Robb amendment (introduced by Senator Charles Robb as amendment 3598 to H.R. 4577); H.R. 4680 (introduced by Representative William Thomas), which passed the

House of Representatives in October 2000; and Breaux-Frist II (S. 2807, introduced by Senator John Breaux). Those four proposals cover a broad spectrum of approaches for delivering a Medicare drug benefit. Each year, when CBO updates its 10-year projections of drug spending by or for Medicare beneficiaries, it also updates its estimates for those proposals as a way to reassess key assumptions used in its estimating models.

One issue surrounding a prescription drug benefit is whether it should be a freestanding addition to Medicare (referred to as a stand-alone benefit) or part of a broad effort to restructure the program. Some policymakers advocate expanding Medicare benefits only as one element of a more-sweeping reform that would change cost-sharing rules, introduce competitive features, and add prescription drug coverage as an integrated benefit.

U.S. demographic pressures mean that without major changes in Medicare's design and financing, the cost of the program will grow dramatically over the next 30 years as the large baby-boom generation becomes eligible for benefits.[1] At the same time, Social Security and Medicaid will face an explosion in costs for the same reason (*see Figure 1*). Consequently, without significant changes, the amount that the federal government spends on those three programs is projected to consume a substantial portion of what it now spends on the entire budget.

Broad proposals to reform Medicare raise issues that go well beyond those raised by proposals for a stand-alone drug benefit. This study does not address those wider issues. Rather, it focuses on several important questions concerning a freestanding drug benefit that would be available to beneficiaries under the present Medicare system, including people enrolled in fee-for-service Medicare or in Medicare+Choice plans. Many policy analysts have argued that fully integrating a drug benefit into Medicare and ensuring stable funding for the program in the future can only be accomplished in the context of

---

1. See the statement of Dan L. Crippen, Director, Congressional Budget Office, "Projections of Medicare and Prescription Drug Spending," before the Senate Committee on Finance, March 7, 2002.

Figure 1.

Spending for Social Security, Medicare, and Medicaid, 2000-2030

(Percentage of GDP)

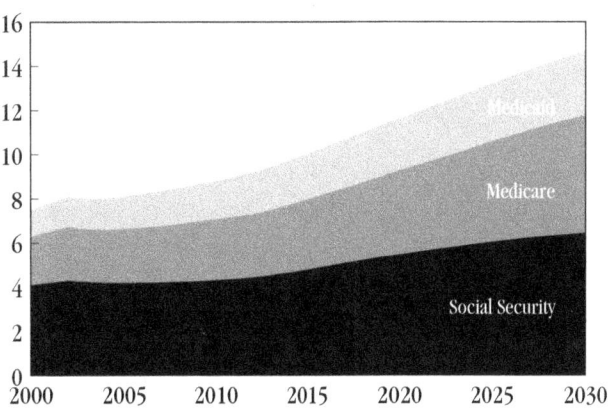

Source: Congressional Budget Office based on its midrange assumptions about growth of gross domestic product and program spending. For further details, see Congressional Budget Office, *The Budget and Economic Outlook: Fiscal Years 2003-2012* (January 2002), Chapter 6.

comprehensive reform. Such reform is an important policy choice but is beyond the scope of this analysis.

Likewise, this study does not discuss other legislative initiatives that relate to prescription drugs but are not directly part of a Medicare drug benefit. For example, under current federal law, manufacturers of brand-name drugs that wish to have their products reimbursed by Medicaid must give that program the best price available to most other purchasers. If the Congress made drug prices for Medicare exempt from that rule, so that Medicare's discounts from drugmakers would not affect Medicaid's best price, then Medicare might be able to negotiate even lower prices. As a result, the cost of a Medicare drug benefit could decline. In addition, changes in policies governing how the Food and Drug Administration regulates such matters as the introduction of new drugs, promotion and advertising for prescription drugs, or reimportation of U.S.-made drugs that were first exported to other countries at lower prices could affect the cost of a Medicare benefit. Although policymakers might consider initiatives in those and other areas as possible ways to save money, each change would raise a host of issues unrelated to a Medicare drug benefit.

1

Medicare Beneficiaries' Drug Spending and Coverage

Several trends are fueling the drive to add a prescription drug benefit to Medicare. Spending for prescription drugs continues to be the fastest growing segment of health care costs. And although Medicare beneficiaries make up nearly 15 percent of the U.S. population, they account for about 40 percent of that spending, which means that increases in drug costs affect them disproportionately. Altogether, Medicare beneficiaries will use nearly $87 billion of outpatient prescription drugs in 2002—an amount that is expected to grow by about 12 percent a year over the next decade (even without a drug benefit in the Medicare program).

In terms of drug coverage, what was traditionally Medicare beneficiaries' main source, employment-based health plans for retirees, has been scaling back benefits in many cases. An additional factor is that Medicare beneficiaries with the highest and lowest income are more likely to have drug coverage (private and public, respectively). People in the low to middle part of the income scale are less likely to have coverage; thus, they pay a higher-than-average proportion of their drug costs from their own pockets.

Nevertheless, the fundamental issue inherent in the debate about adding a drug benefit to Medicare may not be one of providing for use of prescription drugs so much as one of redistributing the cost of drugs away from the people, companies, and government entities that now pay for them. Currently, about three-quarters of Medicare beneficiaries have some kind of insurance to help defray the cost of drugs. The remainder, who have no drug coverage, filled an average of 25 prescriptions in 1999, the Congressional Budget Office estimates, compared with an average of 32 prescriptions for Medicare beneficiaries who have drug coverage.

Beneficiaries' Spending on Prescription Drugs

In recent years, the growth of prescription drug spending has far outpaced the growth of spending for other types of health care. Between 1990 and 2000, for example, annual spending on prescription drugs in the United States grew nearly twice as fast as total national health expenditures (which in turn grew significantly faster than the economy during that period, and continues to do so). Moreover, since the mid-1990s, drug spending has increased at a double-digit rate each year.

For the U.S. population as a whole, three factors explain most of that growth: the introduction of new and costlier drug treatments, broader use of prescription drugs by a larger number of people, and (until recently) lower cost-sharing requirements by private health plans. New brand-name drugs tend to be much more expensive than older drug therapies that treat the same disease. And even as prescription drugs have become more costly, more people have been using them, for several reasons. Many new drugs provide better treatment or have fewer side effects than older alternatives. At the same time, insurance coverage has made such drugs relatively affordable. In addition, more people are aware of new drug therapies through such sources as the Internet and the "direct-to-consumer" advertising campaigns of pharmaceutical manufacturers.

Table 1.

Prescription Drug Spending and Medicare Benefits per Beneficiary, 2003-2012

(By calendar year)

	Spending per Medicare Beneficiary (Dollars)		Average Annual Percentage Change,
	2003	2012	2003-2012
Outpatient Prescription Drugs[a]	2,439	5,816	10.1
Medicare Benefits[b]	6,775	10,794	5.3
Memorandum:			
Gross Domestic Product per Capita	37,900	55,800	4.4

Source: Congressional Budget Office's March 2002 baseline projections.

Note: These numbers assume the continuation of the current Medicare program, with no outpatient prescription drug benefit.

a. Total spending per beneficiary on outpatient prescription drugs not currently covered under Medicare, regardless of payer.

b. Benefits and administrative costs per beneficiary under the Hospital Insurance and Supplementary Medical Insurance programs.

CBO expects prescription drug spending by Medicare beneficiaries (or their health plans) to rise rapidly over the next decade—at an average rate per person of 10.1 percent a year (*see Table 1*).[1] That rate is significantly faster than the projected growth of spending for current Medicare benefits, and more than twice as fast as the expected per capita growth of the U.S. economy. Medicare beneficiaries, employers who offer health coverage for retirees, and state governments have pushed for a Medicare drug benefit to obtain some financial relief from those rising expenditures.

Distribution of Beneficiaries' Drug Spending

Although most Medicare beneficiaries use some prescription drugs, the bulk of drug spending is concentrated among a relatively small group. A large share of that spending pays for the treatment of chronic conditions,

---

1. That estimate assumes the continuation of the current Medicare program, with no outpatient prescription drug benefit.

such as hypertension, cardiovascular disease, and diabetes. The skewed distribution of spending—and the need for people with chronic conditions to stay on drug therapies for a long time—makes voluntary stand-alone drug coverage particularly susceptible to the problem of adverse selection, in which enrollment in an insurance plan is concentrated among people who expect to receive more in benefits than they pay in premiums. (That problem is discussed in detail in Chapter 3.)

CBO projects that prescription drug spending by or for Medicare beneficiaries will total more than $128 billion in 2005 (the first year in which Medicare could probably begin implementing a prescription drug benefit that was enacted in 2002). In that year, about 64 percent of Medicare beneficiaries will spend over $1,000 on prescription drugs, CBO estimates; their combined spending will make up 96 percent of total drug expenditures by Medicare beneficiaries (*see Table 2*). Only 17 percent of beneficiaries are expected to spend more than $5,000 on pre-

Table 2.

Prescription Drug Spending by or for Medicare Beneficiaries, 2005

Spending Level per Beneficiary (Dollars)	Percentage of Beneficiaries with Spending Above That Level[a]	Percentage of Beneficiaries' Total Drug Spending[b]
0	89.8	100.0
500	75.1	98.9
1,000	64.4	96.1
2,000	47.4	87.5
3,000	33.7	75.8
4,000	24.5	64.8
5,000	17.3	53.7
6,000	12.4	44.5
7,000	9.3	37.6
8,000	6.9	31.5
9,000	5.5	27.2
10,000	4.3	23.4

Source: Congressional Budget Office's March 2002 baseline projections.

Note: These numbers do not include spending for outpatient prescription drugs currently covered by Medicare.

a. Total Medicare enrollment for 2005 is projected to be 41.9 million people.

b. Beneficiaries' total spending for outpatient prescription drugs in 2005 is projected to be $128.1 billion.

Figure 2.

Sources of Payment for Medicare Beneficiaries' Prescription Drugs, 1999

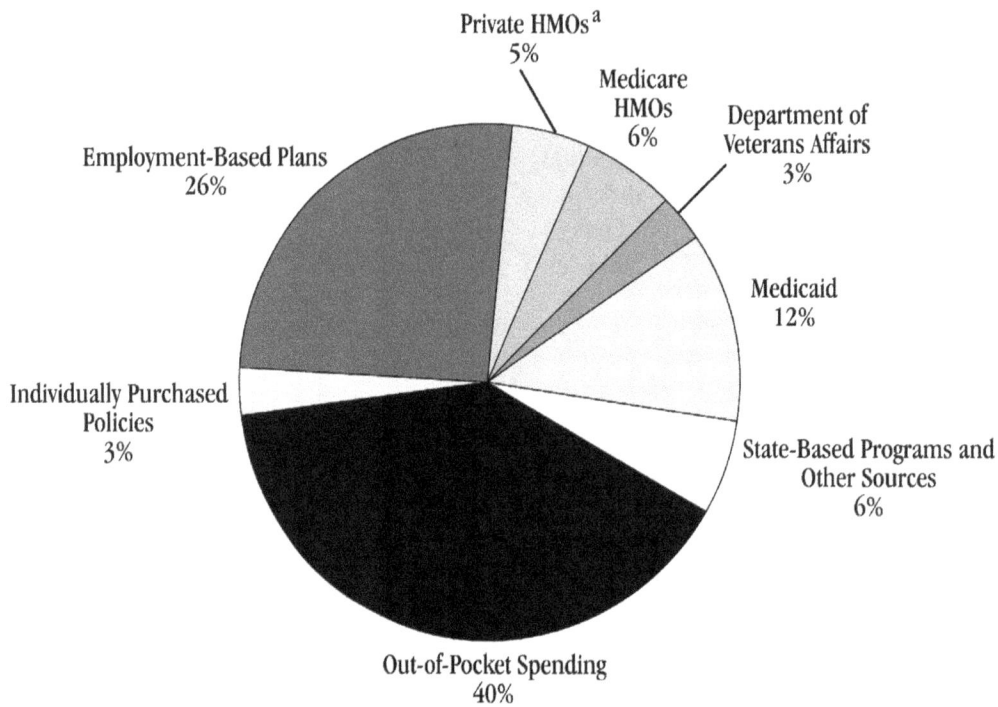

Source: Congressional Budget Office based on data from the 1999 Medicare Current Beneficiary Survey.

Note: HMOs = health maintenance organizations.

a. These are generally also employment-based plans.

scription drugs in 2005, but their spending will make up nearly 54 percent of the total.

Beneficiaries' Existing Drug Coverage

Certain factors suggest that growth in drug spending has a larger financial impact on Medicare beneficiaries than on other segments of the population. On average, 40 percent of Medicare beneficiaries' drug expenditures came from their own pockets in 1999 (the most recent year for which data are available), compared with about 33 percent for the U.S. population as a whole (see Figure 2). Also, because Medicare beneficiaries are elderly or disabled, they are more likely to have chronic health conditions and to use more prescription drugs: nearly 90 percent filled at least one prescription in 1999, compared with just over 60 percent of the population as a whole. Medicare beneficiaries made up nearly 15 percent of the population that year, but they accounted for about

40 percent of spending on outpatient prescription drugs in the United States.

Overall statistics, however, mask a wide variety of personal circumstances. In 1999, one-quarter of the Medicare population had no prescription drug coverage. The other three-quarters of beneficiaries obtained drug coverage as part of a plan that supplemented Medicare's benefits. But those supplemental plans differed greatly in the extent of drug coverage they provided.

Employment-Based Plans

Traditionally, more elderly people have received prescription drug coverage from retiree health plans than from any other source. In 1999, about 30 percent of Medicare beneficiaries had supplemental health insurance through a current or former employer, and most of those health plans covered prescription drugs (see Table 3). Although specific benefits vary, employment-based drug coverage

Table 3.

Medicare Beneficiaries' Prescription Drug Coverage, 1999

Type of Drug Coverage	Number of Medicare Beneficiaries with That Coverage (Millions)	Percentage of All Medicare Beneficiaries	Average Number of Prescriptions Filled
Medicaid[a]	6.4	15.9	39
Employment-Based Plan	11.9	29.6	31
Individually Purchased (Medigap) Policy	4.5	11.2	32
Other Public Coverage[b]	1.7	4.1	37
HMO Not Elsewhere Classified[c]	5.7	14.2	28
Subtotal	30.2	75.0	32
No Drug Coverage	10.1	25.0	25
Total	**40.4**	**100.0**	**30**

Source: Congressional Budget Office based on data from the 1999 Medicare Current Beneficiary Survey.

Note: Some Medicare beneficiaries have more than one type of coverage for outpatient prescription drugs. The categories in this table are mutually exclusive, and CBO assigned people to categories in the order shown above.

a. Beneficiaries who received any Medicaid benefits during the year, including those eligible for a state's full package of benefits (so-called dual eligibles and people who meet eligibility requirements after paying their Medicaid expenses).
b. Beneficiaries who received aid for their drug spending through state-sponsored pharmaceutical assistance programs, the Department of Veterans Affairs, the Department of Defense, or health maintenance organizations under Medicare+Choice nonrisk contracts.
c. Primarily health maintenance organizations under Medicare+Choice risk contracts.

tends to feature relatively low deductibles and copayments.

Many employers have begun to restructure their benefits, however, because prescription drug spending by elderly retirees has become a significant cost. A 1997 study by Hewitt Associates for the Kaiser Family Foundation found that among large employers, drug spending for people age 65 or older constituted 40 percent to 60 percent of the total cost of their retiree health plans.[2] Average use of prescription drugs among elderly retirees was more than double that of current workers. Although relatively few employers in the Hewitt survey had dropped retiree coverage altogether, most had taken steps to control costs, such as tightening eligibility standards, requiring retirees to pay a greater share of their premiums, placing caps on

the amount of benefits that plans will cover, and encouraging elderly beneficiaries to enroll in managed care plans.

Other Sources of Drug Coverage
Another way in which elderly or disabled people can obtain prescription drug coverage is through Medicare+ Choice (M+C) plans. In 2002, 50 percent of Medicare beneficiaries have access to M+C plans that offer some drug coverage. But a far smaller fraction of beneficiaries, about 9 percent, sign up for those plans. In addition, many M+C plans have scaled back their drug benefits in response to higher drug costs and slower growth in Medicare's payment rates. Nearly all such plans have annual caps on enrollees' drug benefits, and a growing percentage charge a premium for supplemental benefits. Some plans limit their coverage to generic drugs, with no coverage for brand-name prescriptions.

About 23 percent of the Medicare population relied on individually purchased (medigap) plans as their main

---

2. Hewitt Associates, Kaiser Medicare Policy Project, *Retiree Health Trends and Implications of Possible Medicare Reforms* (Washington, D.C.: Hewitt Associates, September 1997), available at www.kff. org/content/archive/1318/retiree_r.html.

form of supplemental health coverage in 1999, but less than half of that group had policies that covered prescription drugs. Medigap plans with drug coverage tend to be much less generous than retiree health plans: they have an annual deductible of $250, require cost sharing of 50 percent, and limit yearly benefits to either $1,250 or $3,000. Premiums for medigap plans that include drug coverage also tend to be much higher than premiums for other medigap plans, in part because of their tendency to attract enrollees who have higher-than-average health expenses.

Some low-income Medicare beneficiaries are eligible for Medicaid coverage, which generally includes a prescription drug benefit. All state Medicaid programs offer drug coverage (usually with little or no cost sharing) to people whose income and assets fall below certain thresholds. In addition, as of September 2002, 34 states had authorized (though not necessarily begun implementing) some type of pharmaceutical assistance program. Many of those programs will provide direct aid for drug purchases to low-income elderly people who do not meet the eligibility requirements for Medicaid. In all, about 76 percent of the Medicare population lives in those states.

On average, Medicare beneficiaries with drug coverage had about 32 prescriptions filled in 1999. Those without drug coverage used fewer prescription drugs that year, but they still had an average of 25 prescriptions filled.

Differences by Income Level

Many middle- and higher-income seniors can obtain coverage through retiree plans, and seniors with the lowest income generally have access to state-based drug benefit programs. However, Medicare beneficiaries with income between one and three times the federal poverty level tend to be caught in the middle: they are less likely than poorer seniors to qualify for state assistance and less likely than higher-income seniors to have access to drug coverage through former employers. In 1999, nearly half of Medicare beneficiaries had income between one and three times the poverty level, and almost 30 percent of them had no drug coverage (*see Table 4*). People in those income groups paid more of their drug costs out of pocket than other Medicare beneficiaries did (44 percent versus 34 percent).

Table 4.

Medicare Beneficiaries' Prescription Drug Coverage and Spending, by Income Level, 1999

Income Relative to the Federal Poverty Level	Number of Medicare Beneficiaries (Millions)	Percentage of All Medicare Beneficiaries	Percentage of Income Group Without Drug Coverage	Spending on Outpatient Prescription Drugs (Billions of dollars)	
				Total Spending	Out-of-Pocket Spending
Less Than 100 Percent	6.6	16.2	20.0	8.3	2.0
100 to 200 Percent	11.4	28.2	31.4	13.4	5.8
200 to 300 Percent	8.1	20.1	25.5	9.6	4.2
300 Percent or More	14.3	35.4	22.0	19.3	7.4
Total	**40.4**	**100.0**	**25.0**	**50.5**	**19.4**

Source: Congressional Budget Office based on data from the 1999 Medicare Current Beneficiary Survey.

Note: CBO adjusted each beneficiary's level of drug spending by 25 percent to reflect underreporting in the survey. Prescription drug spending for survey respondents in nursing homes was imputed from the spending of noninstitutionalized respondents who have trouble with the same number of activities of daily living.

2

Design Choices for a Medicare Drug Benefit

In designing a drug benefit for Medicare, policymakers must make four fundamental decisions:

■ How comprehensive will the coverage be?

■ Who will be eligible to enroll?

■ To what extent will the government pay enrollees' costs?

■ How and by whom will the drug program be administered?

The answers to each of those questions will have a major impact on the program's cost to the federal government and to enrollees. (This chapter and the next describe, in general, how various approaches to those choices affect costs. Specific cost estimates for particular proposals are discussed in Chapter 4.)

In addition, most of those decisions will involve trade-offs among the various goals for a Medicare prescription drug benefit. For example, features designed to encourage wide enrollment—such as extensive coverage, low deductibles and copayments, broad eligibility, and subsidies for low-income enrollees—will also make the program more expensive for the federal government (and possibly for state and local governments). But features designed to control costs—such as narrow coverage, high cost sharing by enrollees, and limited eligibility—may mean that fewer Medicare beneficiaries receive the benefits of prescription drug coverage.

Any program in which the federal government subsidizes a large share of drug costs for many enrollees will require substantial federal outlays. Medicare beneficiaries are expected to spend an average of nearly $2,500 apiece on outpatient prescription drugs in 2003. Access to better drug coverage would undoubtedly stimulate further spending. However, decisions about how to administer the drug benefit can exacerbate or alleviate the federal cost burden. Consequently, those decisions are especially important.

All of the recent proposals for a Medicare drug program would rely on private entities to administer the benefit, but there are significant differences in the functions envisioned for those entities. Opportunities exist to manage drug use and prices prudently, but pharmacy benefit managers need both the incentives and the tools to do so. The Congressional Budget Office has concluded that among the designs for a Medicare drug program proposed in the past few years, those with certain administrative features offer the greatest opportunity for constraining federal costs and total spending on outpatient prescription drugs. Although not without shortcomings, those designs have three main features: they allow benefit managers to employ the full array of tools now used to administer private-sector drug plans, they force benefit managers to compete among themselves for enrollees' business, and they make managers assume financial risk for delivering benefits.

Figure 3.

Hypothetical Structure of a Medicare Prescription Drug Benefit

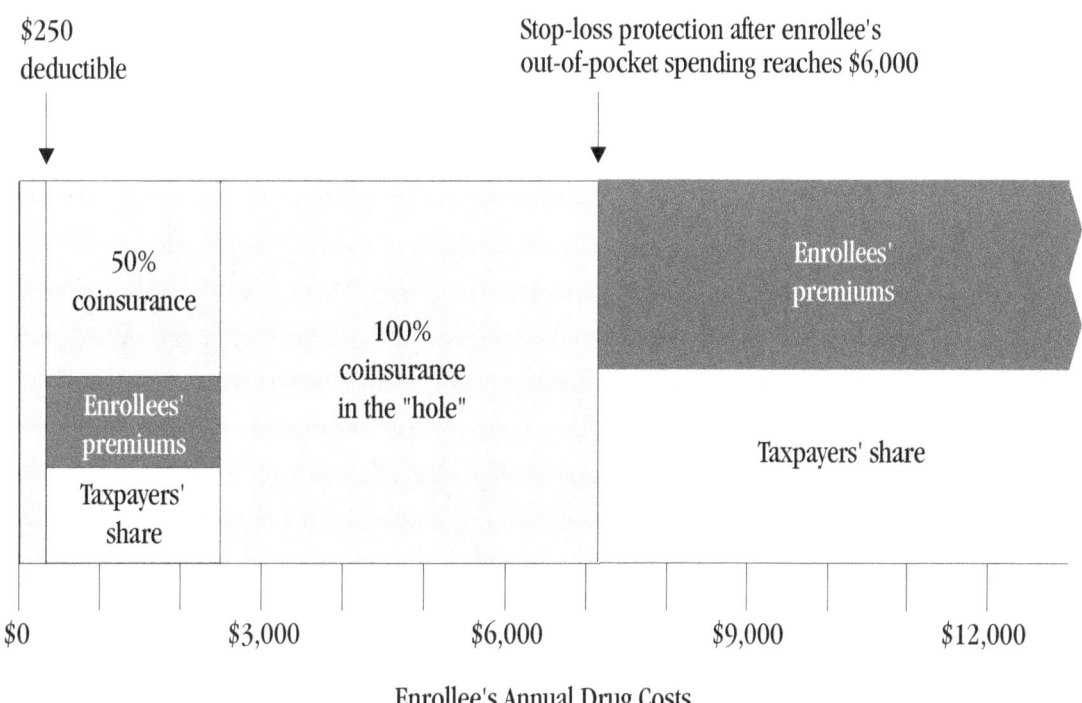

Source: Congressional Budget Office.

The Structure of the Coverage

The single biggest determinant of the cost of a Medicare drug benefit is how the coverage is designed. Choices about the structure of the coverage include:

- The deductible amount (whether coverage begins with the first dollar of drug spending in a given year or after the deductible amount is reached);

- Cost-sharing rates (what share of the cost of a prescription is the responsibility of the enrollee);[1]

- The benefit cap (the level of spending beyond which the enrollee must pay the full cost of each prescription); and

---

1. Cost-sharing rates can be specified as dollar amounts (copayments) or as a percentage of costs (coinsurance).

- The catastrophic stop-loss amount (the level of spending beyond which the enrollee pays little or nothing for prescriptions).

The possible variations on those choices are numerous and could produce benefits unlike anything available in the private sector today. Of the four proposals discussed in Chapter 4, the Clinton Administration's plan and H.R. 4680 both include a capped benefit, then a "hole" (a level of spending at which there would be no drug coverage), and finally a stop-loss provision, beyond which the benefit would pay all drug costs (*see Figure 3*). Plans currently available through employers, by contrast, almost never include such holes in coverage. The larger the range of spending encompassed by the hole, the less costly the program would be—but also the less coverage the benefit would provide.

The structure of the coverage also indirectly affects the cost of the drug program through the out-of-pocket spending it requires of enrollees. Benefits with low cost-sharing rates would encourage enrollees who were newly shielded from paying the full costs of their drugs to use a greater number of—and more expensive—prescriptions. Conversely, higher cost-sharing rates would induce less new drug spending.

Eligibility for Enrollment

A fundamental design choice concerns whether the prescription drug benefit would be available to all Medicare beneficiaries or only some (on the basis of such criteria as income, wealth, or current drug coverage). The cost of the drug program could be reduced by limiting eligibility. However, most recent proposals for Medicare drug coverage would allow all Medicare beneficiaries to enroll, although they would provide much higher subsidies to low-income beneficiaries.

A second choice for policymakers is whether to make enrollment in the benefit voluntary and, if so, with what restrictions. A voluntary drug program that did not limit when and how often an eligible person could enroll would encourage beneficiaries to sign up only when they expected to incur high drug costs and to opt out again when they expected little need for prescription drugs. All of the proposals examined in Chapter 4 would provide a voluntary drug benefit, but they would restrict that choice by giving people only one opportunity to enroll without penalty (when they first became eligible), or by imposing a surcharge on people who delayed enrollment, to reflect the higher costs that such enrollees typically entail. (When the drug program began, however, all Medicare beneficiaries, regardless of age, would have a chance to sign up for the coverage.)

Besides those two restrictions, another way to reduce beneficiaries' incentives to enroll or drop coverage at will would be to couple the drug benefit with Part B of Medicare (Supplementary Medical Insurance). In that case, beneficiaries could choose either Part B plus drug coverage or no Part B and no drug coverage. Because Medicare currently pays 75 percent of Part B benefits, and because enrollment in Part B without penalty is restricted to a brief period after eligibility begins, virtually all Medicare beneficiaries sign up for Part B. Linking the

drug benefit to enrollment in Part B would probably ensure reasonably high participation in the benefit. However, if enrollment in Part B required enrollment in the drug program and the full premium (for Part B plus drugs) rose substantially as a result, some people who would otherwise enroll in Part B might drop that coverage.

The Level and Structure of Federal Subsidies

Two important design choices are how much the federal government would contribute to the cost of drug coverage for Medicare beneficiaries and how such subsidies would be structured. Those design choices have consequences not only for federal costs but also for costs to state and local governments. In addition, the level of subsidy offered to enrollees would have an important effect on people's willingness to take part in the drug program.

Most of the Medicare drug benefits proposed recently in the Congress would provide some level of federal subsidy for all enrollees, but they would still require those enrollees to contribute substantially—through both cost sharing and premiums. To make drug coverage more affordable to low-income Medicare beneficiaries, most proposals would provide a higher federal subsidy for enrollees who met certain eligibility criteria.

Subsidies for All Enrollees

The higher the subsidy, the greater the number of people who would want to enroll in a drug benefit, but also the greater the costs to the federal government. Widespread enrollment is desirable for two reasons: it means that the drug benefit is accomplishing the goal of providing insurance to most Medicare beneficiaries, and it reduces the likelihood that enrollees will be drawn disproportionately from people who expect to have high drug costs. The question for policymakers is, How large would the federal subsidy have to be to induce most Medicare beneficiaries to enroll?

Even if the federal subsidy was small, enrollment would still be fairly high because many people with private or public drug coverage would probably be required to enroll. For example, employment-based health plans would probably require retirees eligible for a Medicare drug benefit to participate in it, just as they now effectively require that retirees participate in Part B. Even employers who offered to pay Medicare's drug premium for retirees would have lower costs so long as that premium was subsidized to any extent (assuming their retirees were not markedly less costly than the average Medicare participant). The more comprehensive Medicare's drug coverage was, the more employers' health care costs for retirees would be reduced, but they would probably take advantage of even a limited drug benefit. Likewise, state Medicaid agencies, even if not required to do so, would choose to enroll people eligible for both Medicare and Medicaid in a Medicare drug program if states' costs under the new program were less than under Medicaid's current drug benefit.

Thus, the people whose participation would be most sensitive to the size of the federal subsidy would be the one-quarter of Medicare beneficiaries without drug coverage from private or public sources. If the drug benefit was not subsidized and enrollment was always open, few of those beneficiaries would be likely to enroll. If, however, they had only one chance to enroll without financial penalty, some of those beneficiaries would probably take part without any federal subsidy, and most would choose to enroll at subsidy rates well below 100 percent of the cost. The reason is that virtually all beneficiaries would expect to receive more in benefits in some years than the premiums they paid. One-time-only enrollment would also increase the extent of participation for any given level of subsidy. However, a drug benefit that was financed mainly by enrollees could be difficult for some people to afford—specifically, people whose income or assets were only slightly too high to qualify for drug coverage through Medicaid or other public programs.

Subsidies for Low-Income Enrollees

Creating an additional subsidy program for low-income users of a Medicare drug benefit requires making decisions about such things as eligibility for the subsidy, the size of the subsidy, and whether states would pay a share. Those choices would affect enrollment in the drug benefit and its cost to the federal government and the states.

Who Would Be Eligible? As noted earlier, some low-income Medicare beneficiaries receive assistance for part or all of their medical costs through the federal/state Medicaid program. Those beneficiaries fall into three categories.

- *Dual eligibles* meet all state requirements for Medicaid eligibility, either because their income and assets are below the limits set by a state or because they have "spent down" their resources to those limits as a result of high medical costs (in which case they are referred to as the medically needy). People in the first group have their Medicare premiums and cost sharing paid by Medicaid. They also receive all Medicaid benefits, including coverage for prescription drugs. Most medically needy beneficiaries receive the same benefits, although a few states do not cover their expenses for drugs.

- *Qualified Medicare beneficiaries* (QMBs) have income below the federal poverty level and meet certain restrictions on financial assets. About 75 percent of them qualify as dual eligibles; the other 25 percent are eligible for benefits only as QMBs. That group has its Medicare premiums and cost sharing paid by Medicaid but is not eligible for other Medicaid benefits, such as drug coverage.

- *Specified low-income Medicare beneficiaries* (SLMBs) have income between 100 percent and 120 percent of the federal poverty level and meet certain restrictions on financial assets. About one-third of them qualify as dual eligibles; the other two-thirds qualify only as SLMBs. The sole benefit that SLMBs receive from Medicaid is payment of their Medicare Part B premiums.

Most proposals for a Medicare drug benefit include some form of low-income subsidy for beneficiaries in all of those categories.

In addition, most recent Medicare drug proposals would assist other low-income Medicare beneficiaries. Proposals typically call for providing subsidies to all enrollees with income below 135 percent of the poverty level (and limited assets), which would cover their premiums and cost sharing for prescription drugs. Enrollees with income between 135 percent and 150 percent of the poverty level would have some or all of their premiums subsidized. Many proposals would extend the subsidies to enrollees with even higher income. (A few proposals would remove limits on assets.)

How Much Would States Pay? A key design choice for low-income subsidies is how much would be funded by the federal government and how much by the states. The federal government now pays 57 percent of Medicaid costs, on average, with the states covering the rest. Some proposals for a Medicare drug benefit would maintain the current federal percentage for dual eligibles and QMBs. However, the federal government would pay the full subsidy for other low-income enrollees (those who met special income and asset limits established for low-income subsidies in the drug program). Other proposals would require the federal government to pay the full cost of the subsidies for all low-income enrollees, including dual eligibles. In many of those cases, states would be required to reimburse the federal government for some share of the amount they saved under the proposal.

A proposal that increased the federal government's share of the cost of low-income subsidies would reduce states' costs, and vice versa. The low-income subsidy would also augment or (at the state's option) replace state-run drug programs for low-income seniors who are not eligible for Medicaid. As noted earlier, 34 states either have introduced or are planning to introduce such programs. A federal subsidy of Medicare beneficiaries in those programs would directly reduce state spending.

Who Would Participate? The cost of a low-income subsidy program would ultimately depend on how many people participated. Not all eligible Medicare beneficiaries would choose to receive a low-income subsidy even if they enrolled in the drug benefit. Some might want to avoid being associated with a government "welfare" program; others might not believe that they were eligible for or needed the subsidy.

What entity was chosen to administer the low-income subsidy program could affect the level of participation. CBO estimates that only 50 percent of people eligible for QMB subsidies and 30 percent of those eligible for SLMB subsidies take part in those programs today. Most recent proposals for a Medicare drug benefit would rely on state Medicaid agencies to determine eligibility and enroll low-income beneficiaries—as the QMB and SLMB programs do now. However, another option would be to have the Social Security Administration (SSA) provide those enrollment services. Participation would be higher under that arrangement because less "welfare" stigma is associated with SSA than with Medicaid.

As was the case with subsidies for all enrollees, the size of the low-income subsidies would also influence participation. A larger subsidy would almost certainly induce more people to take part in the low-income program.

That effect would also depend on the design of the Medicare drug coverage. High deductibles or premiums might persuade eligible low-income beneficiaries to sign up for the low-income subsidy to cover those up-front costs. Similarly, the more generous the coverage of drug expenses beyond the deductible, the stronger would be the incentive to enroll.

Perhaps the major issue affecting participation by low-income beneficiaries is whether the asset standards now in place for Medicaid would be relaxed for the Medicare drug benefit. Most proposals would retain the asset standards currently used to determine QMBs and SLMBs. However, less-stringent standards would expand the number of people eligible for low-income subsidies.

The Effect on Spending for Medicaid. Adding prescription drug coverage to Medicare would alter not only federal spending for that program but also federal and state spending for Medicaid. Such coverage would reduce Medicaid's costs for dual eligibles because Medicare would pick up part of their prescription drug costs. However, some of that reduction would be offset by higher enrollment in the Medicaid program. Some people who are now eligible for Medicaid do not enroll; a Medicare drug benefit would give them a new incentive to do so, because under most proposals, state Medicaid programs would administer the low-income subsidies. Thus, people applying for Medicare drug coverage under the low-income subsidy would learn about their eligibility for Medicaid and enroll in that program at the same time.

Other Factors Affecting the Cost of Low-Income Subsidies. The effect on federal costs for low-income subsidies would depend not just on the factors discussed above but also on the interplay between the coverage provided by a Medicare drug benefit and the provisions for low-income subsidies. In general, increasing cost sharing for enrollees in the drug benefit would lead to higher federal subsidies for low-income enrollees. Conversely, reducing enrollees' cost sharing would result in lower federal costs for low-income subsidies.

Administrative Approach

The way in which a Medicare drug program was administered could also have a significant impact on its cost. Most recent proposals envision the approach—now common in the private sector—of using organizations such as pharmacy benefit managers (PBMs) to administer the benefit. The proposals differ, however, in the number of such organizations that would serve a region, the restrictions they would be subject to, the basis on which they could compete for enrollees, and whether they would assume any insurance risk. (Insurance risk occurs when the entity providing coverage is liable for payments that may not be fully covered by premiums or reimbursements or, conversely, is allowed to keep part of surpluses when costs fall short of premiums or reimbursements.)

In the past decade, PBMs have come to play a central role in administering prescription drug benefits in the private sector (*see Figure 4*). Their main function is to act as a health plan's agent in administering a drug benefit. PBMs do not distribute prescription drugs to patients, except when they own mail-order or community pharmacies. Instead, prescription drugs flow from manufacturers to dispensing pharmacies (often with stops along the way at wholesalers' warehouses) and then to consumers, either at pharmacies or by mail. A pharmacy pays a manufacturer for the drugs it purchases and in turn charges a price it

has negotiated with the PBM. The consumer and health plan share the responsibility for paying that price.

PBMs perform various functions and use various management tools. They process and pay claims. On behalf of a health plan and its enrollees, they also negotiate price discounts with dispensing pharmacies and rebates with drug manufacturers. In return for receiving rebates, PBMs try to steer enrollees toward preferred or formulary drugs. (A formulary is a list of drugs that the health plan will cover. Nonpreferred drugs are covered and therefore included in the formulary, but they typically entail higher cost sharing for the enrollee than preferred drugs do.) PBMs' other strategies for lowering costs include encouraging the use of generic drugs and dispensing drugs through mail-order pharmacies, which many large PBMs own. PBMs may establish and enforce differential cost-sharing requirements to encourage enrollees to select lower-cost drugs. In addition, because they keep centralized records of each enrollee's prescriptions, they can help prevent inappropriate dosages and harmful drug interactions.[2]

Although PBMs in the private sector often have considerable leeway in the tools they can use, they do not assume any insurance risk for the drug benefits they administer. However, they may have a bonus added to, or a penalty subtracted from, their administrative fee on the basis of how well they meet preset goals for their performance.

Some of the Medicare drug proposals developed during the 106th Congress, such as the Clinton Administration's, called for a single PBM selected periodically to serve each region, with all insurance risk borne by Medicare, not the PBM. Other proposals, such as H.R. 4680, adopted a different approach: they would use multiple risk-bearing entities (such as PBM/insurer partnerships) that would compete to serve enrollees in each region. En-

---

2. See, for example, E.P. Armstrong and C.R. Denemark, "How Pharmacists Respond to On-Line, Real-Time DUR Alerts," *Journal of the American Pharmaceutical Association*, vol. 38, no. 2 (March-April 1998), pp. 149-154; and Stephen Soumerai and Helene Lipton, "Computer-Based Drug-Utilization Review," *New England Journal of Medicine*, vol. 332, no. 24 (June 15, 1995), pp. 1641-1645.

Figure 4.

The Role of PBMs in the Flow of Money and Prescription Drugs

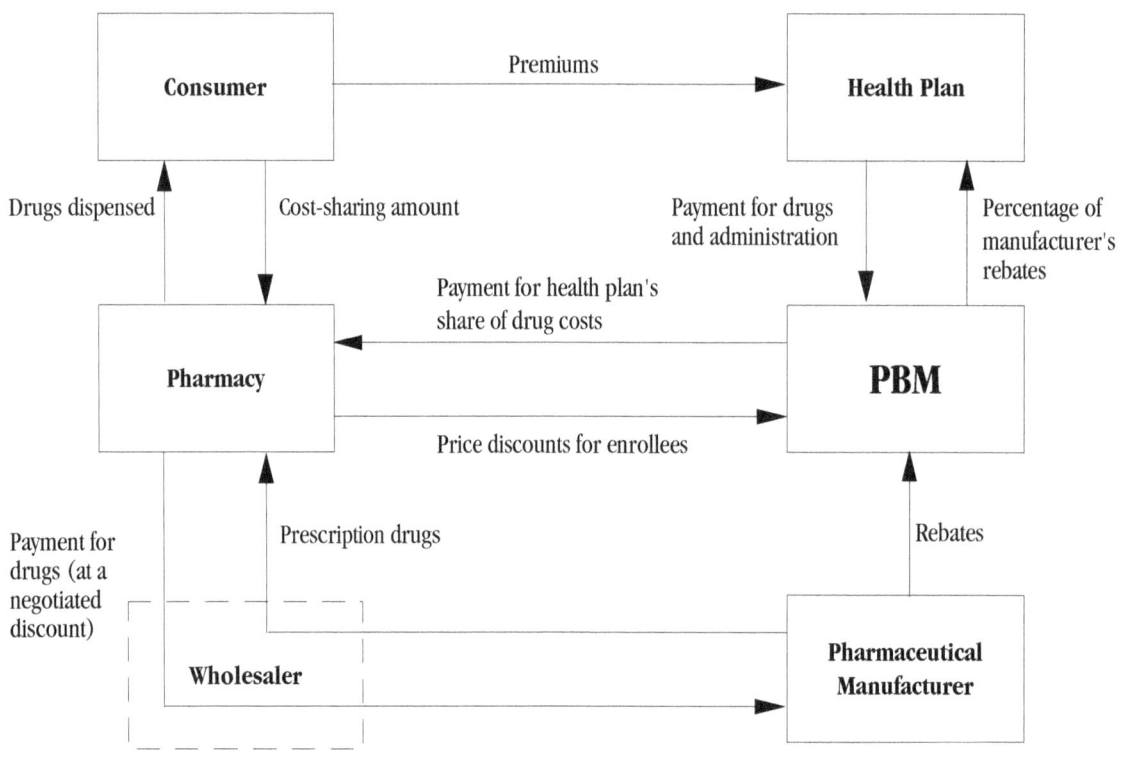

Source: Congressional Budget Office.

Note: PBM = pharmacy benefit manager.

rollees would have some choice among entities, so people who were willing to accept more restrictive rules (such as a limited formulary) in return for lower cost sharing or premiums could do so, while others could select a more expensive plan with fewer restrictions. Hybrid models have been proposed in which multiple entities would compete for enrollees without bearing insurance risk. They could compete on the basis of such features as lower drug prices, fewer limits on covered drugs, and wider networks of pharmacies.

Each administrative model has its pros and cons. The next chapter describes how each model addresses key problems inherent in designing a Medicare prescription drug program—such as the risk to plans from enrolling a disproportionately large share of people with high expected drug costs, the need to control drug spending, and the feasibility of administering the benefit efficiently.

3
Problems in Designing a Medicare Drug Benefit

Although the choices available to policymakers seem numerous, many proposals for a Medicare prescription drug benefit have certain similarities. The reason is that they are trying to address specific problems that arise in designing such a benefit. Those problems include the possibility that the coverage will mainly attract people with the highest drug costs, the need to constrain total costs to the government and to enrollees, the ability and willingness of private entities (such as pharmacy benefit managers) to administer the drug benefit, and the possible side effects of the drug program on other parts of Medicare.

Selection Issues

Policies that would provide stand-alone prescription drug benefits may be especially prone to the insurance-market phenomenon known as adverse selection, in which people who expect to have higher-than-average costs disproportionately enroll in an insurance plan. Adverse selection becomes an issue when plans (or potential enrollees) make decisions based on the desire to avoid attracting (or being grouped with) enrollees who are likely to have expensive claims. For example, the threat of adverse selection may lead insurers to design or manage their plans in such a way as to discourage people with high expected claims from joining. Or they may market their plans in ways that will avoid such enrollees. Similarly, potential enrollees would prefer not to be put in an insurance pool with people who were likely to have high costs, because that

would imply higher premiums than would otherwise be the case. Thus, the potential for adverse selection might cause some people to opt out of insurance altogether.

Adverse selection can occur in an insurance market if subgroups of potential enrollees can be expected to use benefits at a rate that will differ substantially from that of other groups. In the case of prescription drugs, demand is strongly related to whether a person has a chronic medical condition. Thus, many Medicare beneficiaries may have a good idea of their likely drug spending in the short run and, in some cases, even in the long run. If the plan (or plans) that offered Medicare drug coverage could not distinguish between enrollees with high or low expected costs—or was not permitted to treat such enrollees differently in terms of benefits offered or premiums charged—then adverse selection could occur in a voluntary drug program.

Why Is Adverse Selection a Problem?

Adverse selection poses difficulties in several ways. It undermines the purpose of health insurance, which is to spread among a pool of people the financial risks that would arise if some of them developed medical problems. Adverse selection raises the cost of insurance for people who do enroll. And it makes people who do not enroll worse off by not receiving the benefits of insurance. (Even people who anticipate having low medical costs could benefit from insuring against the possibility that they develop an unexpected illness.)

In private insurance markets, adverse selection can create a pattern of high premiums and low enrollment, resulting in much less coverage than would otherwise have been the case.[1] The history of private medigap policies that cover outpatient prescription drugs is a case in point. A variety of insurers sell medigap policies to Medicare beneficiaries who typically lack other sources of supplementary coverage. Since 1992, insurers have been allowed to market only 10 standardized medigap policies, and an insurer must charge the same premium for a given policy to all beneficiaries who enroll when they first become eligible for Medicare. Premiums can rise with a policyholder's age but cannot vary according to his or her health status. Three of the 10 medigap policies available to Medicare beneficiaries include some coverage of prescription drugs. However, that coverage is limited by benefit caps. Even so, those plans are costly compared with medigap plans that exclude drugs.[2] Most experts agree that the reason for the higher costs is that people who buy the drug policies are more likely to use prescription drugs than people who

do not.[3] Today, only 8 percent of Medicare beneficiaries with standardized medigap policies are enrolled in any of the three plans that provide drug coverage.[4]

Two kinds of adverse selection can affect the operation of a Medicare drug benefit: adverse selection into the drug program as a whole, and, if multiple plans are allowed to administer the drug benefit in the same region and bear financial risk for their costs, adverse selection among those plans.

Adverse Selection Into the Overall Drug Program

If relatively healthy Medicare beneficiaries (such as those with no chronic conditions) tended to opt out of drug coverage, the result would be higher per capita costs and premiums for enrollees than would be the case if the benefit covered a representative mix of Medicare beneficiaries. Moreover, if people could enroll or unenroll in the drug program at any time, some would go from paying no premium when healthy (and paying drug expenses out of pocket if an acute condition developed) to enrolling and paying a high premium when they developed a condition requiring treatment with prescription drugs.[5] Such

---

1. In an extreme situation, adverse selection can lead to the absence of an insurance market for some types of risks. For example, in the individual insurance market, health plans will not cover people who have been diagnosed with certain conditions (or will not cover services for those conditions) even though they could charge such people a higher premium; see Joseph P. Newhouse, "Reimbursing Health Plans and Health Providers: Efficiency in Production Versus Selection," *Journal of Economic Literature*, vol. 34 (September 1996), pp. 1236-1263. Researchers have constructed models of the insurance market in which, given the choice between a managed care plan and a fee-for-service plan, more people join the managed care plan than would do so in the absence of selection issues. That happens because the relative premiums of the two types of plans are affected by the health risks of the people who join the plans. If healthier people, on average, prefer a managed care plan, that plan's premiums will be lower than they would have been solely on the basis of any efficiency advantage of the managed care plan. See Roger Feldman and Bryan Dowd, "Risk Segmentation: Goal or Problem?" *Journal of Health Economics*, vol. 19 (2000), pp. 499-512.

2. Lauren A. McCormack and others, "Medigap Reform Legislation of 1990: Have the Objectives Been Met?" *Health Care Financing Review*, vol. 18, no. 1 (Fall 1996), pp. 157-174.

3. People with drug coverage may have higher drug spending than other people for two reasons: adverse selection and the utilization effect of insurance (known as moral hazard in the economics literature). The utilization effect refers to people's greater willingness to spend money on something, such as prescription drugs, when the price they pay has been lowered because of their insurance. The literature on medigap coverage has emphasized adverse selection as the more important reason for high drug spending in medigap policies that cover prescription drugs.

4. See General Accounting Office, *Medigap Insurance: Plans Are Widely Available but Have Limited Benefits and May Have High Costs*, GAO-01-941 (July 2001). That estimate does not include the 40 percent of existing medigap policies that either were issued before benefits were standardized in 1992 or are otherwise exempt from the federal standards. Some of those older policies include prescription drug coverage.

5. Even with some adverse selection, however, the drug benefit could still offer a significant degree of insurance as long as the frequency with which a person could enroll or unenroll was limited in some way. Future medical costs can rarely be predicted accurately, so a drug benefit would help insure against uncertainty even for enrollees with chronic illnesses.

behavior would undermine the value of health insurance, which depends on collecting premiums from people while they are healthy so that enough funds are available to pay the bills of people who face medical expenses.

Paradoxically, although adverse selection into the drug program would increase costs per enrollee, it would most likely reduce the total cost of the drug benefit, because the number of participants would be so much smaller. Such a situation could become unstable, however, with premiums continuing to grow and enrollment continuing to drop.

A number of strategies exist to offset the effects of adverse selection into the drug program by encouraging many people to participate. First, and perhaps most effective, would be requiring one-time enrollment. A "choose it or lose it" policy would foster high participation because even healthy Medicare beneficiaries might be concerned enough about developing an expensive medical condition later on that they would take advantage of a one-time opportunity to enroll. Participation might be further increased by making enrollment in the program automatic unless the beneficiary took action to reject drug coverage.

A second way to limit adverse selection would be to provide substantial government subsidies for the drug benefit. Because people are generally averse to risk, they are willing to buy insurance even if the premiums they pay exceed the value of the claims they expect to file over the length of the policy. (People who are more risk averse than the norm will be willing to pay even more in premiums for a policy with a given expected payout.) A government subsidy would increase the likelihood that a person would receive insurance benefits in excess of his or her premiums, so that person would be more likely to sign up for a policy. Thus, if the government paid, say, 30 percent of an enrollee's premium for drug coverage, even relatively healthy Medicare beneficiaries might find it advantageous to join a pool of less-healthy enrollees if their premium reflected only 70 percent of such costs. And, of course, the greater the number of healthy enrollees who joined, the lower that premium would become.

A third way to address adverse selection is by adjusting premiums for individuals' differences in expected risk (a practice known as risk rating, which is used in many types of insurance).[6] If healthy enrollees were charged a lower premium that reflected their expected cost to the drug program, they would be more likely to join. However, adjusting the premiums that enrollees pay according to their risk of high spending has not been part of Medicare policy or of any recent proposal for a Medicare drug benefit.[7]

Some observers would argue that it would be unfair to charge higher premiums to enrollees whose drug costs were expected to be high because of preexisting medical conditions.[8] Also, some people might argue that Medicare is a form of social insurance that is intended to insure against changes in health status that occur before people reach the eligibility age for Medicare. In that view, everyone joining Medicare when they first become eligible should face the same premium, regardless of their health

---

6. In this study, "risk rating" generally refers to charging people different premiums on the basis of differences in their expected costs. Such differential premiums could be determined when people first enrolled in a plan, on the basis of their health status and history, or could result from periodic adjustments to their premiums based on their claims experience (a practice known as "experience rating"). Those two approaches are not mutually exclusive.

7. Medicare does charge higher premiums to people who decline enrollment in Part B and later decide to join. That policy is intended to strongly discourage people from enrolling only when they are about to face a large medical bill. By contrast, the risk-rated premiums described above are not surcharges for late enrollment but rather differential premiums that would be charged to enrollees when they were first eligible to join, with limited adjustments over time.

8. Other observers have pointed out the inherent subjectivity in fairness arguments. Mark Pauly asks whether it is reasonable for a relatively healthy lower-middle-income person to subsidize a sickly rich person, which is an implication of charging all enrollees the same premium. Pauly suggests that other ways may exist to subsidize sickly people besides requiring uniform premiums. See Mark V. Pauly, "Is Cream-Skimming a Problem for the Competitive Medical Market?" *Journal of Health Economics*, vol. 3, no. 1 (March 1984), pp. 87-95.

status.[9] Also, if Medicare policy allowed people's premiums to vary over time as their health condition or claims costs changed, enrollees would be denied the benefit of being insured against such changes—a benefit that exists when a plan must charge the same premium to everyone. However, enrollees would still be insured against unexpected needs for prescription drugs that arose during the period over which the premium was fixed.

A fourth way to reduce adverse selection would be to make the drug program a mandatory part of Medicare Part B. If drug coverage was incorporated into the broader range of Medicare health benefits, even people who expected to have low drug costs would be inclined to enroll in order to insure against the general medical costs they might face.

Adverse Selection Among Drug Plans

Proposals for a prescription drug benefit that call for competing plans, each facing insurance risk for the claims they pay, can result in interplan adverse selection.[10] That type of adverse selection occurs when beneficiaries with high expected drug costs enroll in certain plans (and avoid others) because they find the design of the coverage or the services offered by certain plans to be particularly appealing (or because the behavior of some insurers discourages them from enrolling in other plans). Interplan adverse selection is likely to exist in two main instances: when plans cannot easily identify potential enrollees with low expected drug costs versus those with high expected

costs; and when, even if they can make that identification, plans are not allowed (or find it costly) to charge different premiums to enrollees on the basis of different expected costs.

Recent proposals that envision multiple at-risk plans competing for enrollees in the same market would require each plan to charge all of its enrollees in that market the same premium, thus making the problems associated with interplan adverse selection more likely. Requiring a plan to charge a uniform premium (often called community rating) may be justified on the grounds that the purpose of health plans is to insure people against medical problems over long periods of time (perhaps even against problems that occurred before they were covered by a plan). The alternative practice, allowing adjustments to premiums through risk rating, may be impractical and would reduce the value of insurance protection.[11]

The potential for interplan adverse selection would be even greater if the government set a single premium for all of the at-risk plans in a region instead of allowing each plan to set its own premium (even if it had to charge that premium to all of its enrollees). In the latter case, a plan that appealed disproportionately to enrollees with higher expected costs could charge a bigger premium to make up for those costs. For their part, higher-cost enrollees might be willing to pay that premium if they found the services or coverage of the plan sufficiently more attractive than those of alternative plans. If, instead, the government set a single premium for all plans, that safety valve for plans would not be available. As a result, plans would be more likely to engage in behavior aimed at avoiding adverse selection (by encouraging favorable selection), unless the government took steps to prevent it.[12]

How Competing Plans Respond to the Risk of Adverse Selection. When adverse selection appears likely, insurers have various ways to avoid enrolling people who are apt

---

9. In some cases, one person may have a history of higher medical costs than another person not because of poorer health but because of a greater inclination to seek medical care. It may be reasonable to charge a higher premium to someone who has shown a greater willingness to use medical treatment for a given health status. In practical terms, however, it would be difficult to separate medical spending that reflected differences in health status from spending that reflected a greater tendency to seek treatment.

10. More generally, the difficulties associated with interplan adverse selection can arise if those plans have a financial stake in keeping per capita claims costs down. That could happen under proposals in which plans did not assume a pure insurance role. For example, if a plan's administrative fee would be reduced or forfeited when the plan exceeded some performance standard that was highly correlated with per capita claims costs, the issue of interplan adverse selection would be a problem.

---

11. Administrative costs would probably limit risk rating even if plans were legally permitted to charge differential premiums. In that case, plans might develop a *limited* number of rates tied to previous claims or specific health conditions.

12. Favorable selection is disproportionate enrollment by people with low expected costs.

to prove unprofitable. One obvious strategy is for plans to aim their marketing at subgroups of the elderly whom they expect to be relatively healthy. Marketing a plan aggressively at golf clubs but not at nursing homes, for example, might reach low-cost enrollees while avoiding high-cost ones.

Medicare drug plans would probably also design their benefit packages in ways that would appeal to relatively healthy enrollees rather than people with high expected costs. They might cap benefits at levels below those likely to be reached by seniors who have chronic conditions that are associated with high drug costs, or they might require substantial cost sharing. They could also use restrictive formularies to tailor their plan's appeal to people who expect to have low drug costs.

In the competition for enrollees with low expected costs, plans might end up offering similar insurance policies and, to discourage high-cost enrollees, might offer the minimum benefit permitted. But even having similar policies would not completely erase the risk of adverse selection or discourage plans from trying to achieve favorable selection, because plans could adopt many different approaches to vary the quantity, quality, and price of the services they offered. Thus, each plan would remain uncertain about the impact of its own and its rivals' approaches on the pool of enrollees it would attract.

Because plans might try to avoid unprofitable enrollees by offering sparse benefits, premiums could well be lower than they would be without the risk of interplan adverse selection. Nevertheless, those premiums would probably still be higher relative to the benefits offered than would otherwise be the case. The reason is that plans might respond to the uncertainty of adverse selection by charging higher premiums, which they could use to accumulate reserve assets to cover unexpectedly high claims. In general, plans' fears of adverse selection are likely to be greatest in the early years of a Medicare drug benefit, as plans learn how enrollees respond to their options and what packages their competitors are offering.

Another result of adverse selection among plans could be an unstable insurance market, in which plans that initially achieved favorable selection would have lower costs and

premiums than plans that experienced adverse selection, causing enrollees to migrate from higher-cost to lower-cost plans.

Ways to Prevent Interplan Adverse Selection. The government could employ various policy tools to mitigate the negative effects of interplan adverse selection: standardizing plans' benefits, standardizing their marketing, or compensating plans for their differential costs through reinsurance or risk adjustment. In addition, as noted above, the government could allow drug plans to charge risk-rated premiums. However, mechanisms that would reduce adverse selection might create other problems.

Standardized Benefits. One strategy would be to require all competing plans to offer certain features. Standardizing deductibles, cost sharing, benefit caps, and other aspects of coverage, for example, would keep plans from using those features as agents of selection. But standardizing benefits might not prevent all selection-related behavior. Plans could use restrictive formularies and other management tools to deter enrollees with high expected costs from choosing them. Virtually all recent legislative proposals have tried to prevent such behavior by requiring plans that use formularies to offer at least one drug in every therapeutic class. (Some proposals have required that plans offer two or more drugs in each class.)

Standardizing benefits could introduce other drawbacks: for instance, the benefit design that was written into regulations might not encourage cost-effective use of the various drugs that are available. Likewise, standardization could stifle innovations in benefit design that might bring about more cost-effective use of prescription drugs. Also, consumers would lose the opportunity to find a plan tailored to their preferences for financial risk or their willingness to face a limited choice of drugs or pharmacies in exchange for lower premiums.

Standardized Marketing. Another possible means to reduce adverse selection is to standardize the ways in which competing entities market their drug plans. Requiring all plans to use similar marketing materials and to have the same procedure for enrolling beneficiaries could prevent plans from targeting their marketing efforts toward consumers who are expected to have lower costs. However, standardized marketing materials could also make differences in coverage more apparent, which (in the absence of standardized benefits) might give plans more incentive to avoid designs that were likely to appeal to enrollees with high expected costs.

Reinsurance. Another way to counter adverse selection is for the government to provide reinsurance to participating plans. (Reinsurance involves a second insurer—in this case, the federal government—assuming some or all of the first insurer's risk.) Under one type of reinsurance mechanism, a drug plan would receive government funds on the basis of the level of claims incurred by each of its enrollees. If an enrollee's claims in a year reached a specific level, the government would pay the plan a certain fraction of the enrollee's additional claims costs. That fraction would increase as the enrollee's claims grew. A schedule of rising marginal reinsurance payments to plans would reduce incentives for selection because plans would receive higher subsidy rates for enrollees who incurred greater drug costs.

Reinsurance payments could also be based on a plan's average claims cost for all enrollees. Only those plans whose average cost exceeded some threshold amount would receive reinsurance payments to cover part or all of that cost. Neither kind of reinsurance would eliminate the possibility of adverse selection, but they would cushion its financial effects on plans and therefore reduce its costs.

Because reinsurance would be retrospective (based on incurred claims), however, it would have an important disadvantage: it would weaken incentives for drug plans to control spending. A plan that controlled costs more effectively would receive a lower proportional federal subsidy because its enrollees would be less likely to reach the spending thresholds that trigger reinsurance subsidies. As a result, reinsurance might reward inefficiency by covering a portion of plans' high costs no matter what the cause.

Risk-Adjustment Mechanisms. The government could also avoid interplan adverse selection by using risk-adjustment mechanisms. Under such a mechanism, the government would pay additional money to plans that enrolled a disproportionate number of people with medical conditions

or other characteristics (such as age) associated with higher drug costs. Ideally, such a mechanism would offer additional payments that were large enough to neutralize plans' incentives to avoid enrollees who were expected to have high drug costs.

Unlike reinsurance, a risk-adjustment mechanism would be prospective rather than retrospective. In other words, it would base the government's payments to plans on likely claims rather than actual claims. Ideally, those payments would be determined in part by measures of an enrollee's health status that were considered good predictors of future drug costs. However, developing an effective risk-adjustment mechanism is still a work in progress. (For more details, *see Box 1.*)

Risk Rating. A system that allowed plans to charge different premiums according to each enrollee's experience with, or likelihood of, claims could also reduce plans' incentives to avoid high-cost enrollees. However, as noted above, such risk-rated premiums dilute the degree to which an insurance plan protects enrollees from uncertainty about their financial liability over the long run.

Policymakers might want to devise a subsidy scheme to cushion the effects of higher premiums on enrollees who were categorized as having high expected costs. A risk-adjusted premium subsidy by the government would be a way of implementing experience rating without demanding higher premiums from enrollees.

If potential enrollees can judge their expected claims better than health plans can, even risk rating of premiums may not be enough to eliminate adverse-selection behavior. The reason is that plans might not be able to determine the premium differentials they would need to charge to protect themselves against attracting enrollees who turned out to be more costly than expected.

Cost Containment

With Medicare beneficiaries expected to use nearly $87 billion of outpatient prescription drugs this year—and that amount projected to grow by about 12 percent per year—adding subsidized drug coverage to Medicare would represent a major financial commitment for the

Box 1.

The Feasibility of Risk Adjusting the Drug Benefit in Competitive Plans

Risk adjustment is a method for varying payments to a health plan according to the expected variation in health care costs among the plan's beneficiaries. (In the case of a Medicare drug benefit, those payments would come from the federal government.) Payment rates are set on the basis of a beneficiary's risk status before each enrollment period begins. Risk adjustment reduces the incentive that plans have to avoid enrolling people who are likely to incur high health care costs.

Risk adjustment is used in some private-sector health insurance plans and in Medicare's payments to Medicare+Choice plans.[1] However, a proven risk-adjustment mechanism does not yet exist for prescription drugs, although researchers are working to create one. For such a mechanism to be successful, it would have to be able to predict an enrollee's future drug costs with a high degree of accuracy. Moreover, it would need to use predictors whose values could not be changed by the actions of a health plan. For example, if a risk-adjustment method relied on a person's past use of health services to predict future use, plans would have less incentive to control their enrollees' drug spending.

Most risk-adjustment methods available today (for predicting the use of health services other than drugs) depend on data about a person's previous use of services.[2] Even then, the available methods predict only a small part of the variation in different people's use of services.[3]

It might be possible to develop a more accurate risk-adjustment method for prescription drugs than for other health services (especially hospital care), because people's drug spending is more stable from year to year. In addition, there would not be the long lag in data collection that exists for other Medicare claims; data on drug utilization would be available more quickly through the electronic claims technology developed by pharmacy benefit managers. Still, by giving plans that did less to manage drug utilization a higher risk score for their enrollees, a risk-adjustment method based on use could undermine incentives for cost control.

Integrating risk adjustment into the design of a Medicare drug benefit would require finding a way to make additional payments to plans for high-cost enrollees on a prospective basis. One approach would be to adjust the government's share of the plan's premium, similar to the approach now used in the Medicare+Choice program. Another method would be to provide "risk" subsidies using an administrative mechanism similar to the one that would be used to provide low-income subsidies to drug plans.

Another issue is how additional risk-adjustment payments would be counted in reaching reinsurance thresholds (in proposals that call for reinsurance). Thresholds could be raised to take such payments into account. The thresholds could be different for different diagnoses or could be applied to a plan's total costs rather than to costs for individuals. As risk adjustment was refined over time, reinsurance payments could be phased out.

---

1. For a review of risk-adjustment methods, see Robert Wood Johnson Foundation, Changes in Health Care Financing and Organization Program, *Risk Adjustment: A Key to Changing Incentives in the Health Insurance Market* (Washington, D.C.: Alpha Center, March 1997), available at http://hcfo.net/pdf/riskreport.pdf.

2. The risk-adjustment method in place for Medicare+Choice plans during the 2000-2003 period is called the principal inpatient diagnostic cost group method. That method identifies high-cost beneficiaries for a year on the basis of the principal inpatient diagnosis assigned to them during an inpatient hospital stay the previous year. The statistical relationship between that diagnosis and total spending on Medicare services the following year is used to calculate a risk score for the beneficiary. Thus, an assignment of elevated risk depends on a patient's entering a hospital. In 2004, the Medicare+Choice program will move to a risk-adjustment method that uses data from outpatient hospital and physician visits as well as from inpatient hospital stays.

That method will continue to assign risk scores that are based on the relationship between a diagnosis and total spending on Medicare services the following year.

3. For a recent comparison of methods for assigning health risks, see Robert B. Cumming and others, *A Comparative Analysis of Claims-Based Methods of Health Risk Assessment for Commercial Populations* (Schaumburg, Ill.: Society of Actuaries, May 2002), available at www.soa.org/sections/riskadjfinal/report1.pdf.

federal government. Indeed, the four proposals discussed in Chapter 4 would cost the government between $195 billion and $512 billion during their first eight years, the Congressional Budget Office estimates. Moreover, Medicare spending is expected to soar over the next three decades as the baby-boom generation becomes eligible for the program.

For all of those reasons, controlling costs is a key problem in designing a Medicare drug benefit. The size of that problem depends on the extent of the benefits offered under the drug program.

As noted earlier, the level of coverage that is provided is the most important determinant of the overall cost of the benefit. The main reason is that more-generous coverage shifts more of the burden of paying for drugs from the consumer to the drug plan. Another reason is that by lowering the effective price that people must pay for a prescription, new or better drug coverage encourages enrollees to use more, or more costly, drugs than they would otherwise. The more extensive the coverage (the lower the deductible, the required cost sharing, and the catastrophic stop-loss limit), the greater the stimulus to demand for prescription drugs—and the greater the burden on cost management to restrict that growth in demand.

The effect of the Medicare benefit on drug spending would depend not only on the structure of the benefit but also on the drug coverage that enrollees receive now—and might continue to receive—from other sources. For the one-quarter of Medicare beneficiaries without drug coverage, demand for prescription drugs would surely rise when they enrolled in the program because they would be paying less for at least some of their drugs. The size of that increase in demand would depend directly on the structure of the benefit.

For the three-quarters of beneficiaries who already have some public or private drug coverage, the effect on their use of prescription drugs would be more complicated. Their demand would increase only if Medicare's benefit was more comprehensive than, or was supplemented by, the coverage they now have. If the Medicare benefit was less comprehensive than their current coverage, their demand for drugs could decline, but only if the Medicare

benefit completely replaced all other coverage. (For more details of how different kinds of supplemental coverage would interact with a Medicare drug benefit, *see Box 2*).

Active management of the Medicare drug benefit could encourage the use of fewer or less-costly drugs. Most recent proposals assume that the benefit would be administered by entities that have the capabilities of pharmacy benefit managers, which most employment-based health plans use to administer and manage their prescription drug benefits. In recent years, private-sector health plans have increasingly refined their cost-sharing rules so that enrollees are encouraged to buy less-expensive drugs and to fill prescriptions through pharmacies in their network or through mail-order facilities (when that form of dispensing is more efficient).

The degree to which PBMs or other entities could effectively control Medicare drug costs would depend on their having both the authority and the incentive to aggressively use the various tools at their disposal. Key among those cost-management tools are formularies and related approaches to steer demand for drugs to preferred products. (For a description of some of those approaches used in the private sector, see Appendix A.)

In addition, requiring benefit managers to assume some insurance risk for the benefits they pay out and allowing multiple entities to compete for enrollees on the basis of premiums and reimbursements would give managers greater incentive to use the tools they have at hand to hold down spending (although both of those approaches would entail some costs). Even the most effective benefit management, however, would not keep the prices of some drugs from rising under a Medicare drug program.

Cost-Management Tools

In general, a trade-off exists between enrollees' ability to easily obtain the drugs of their choice and a plan's effectiveness at managing drug spending. Aggressive use of formularies, preferred-drug systems, generic-pricing systems, pharmacy networks, mail-order pharmacies (when they are less costly), disease management, and physician and patient education can alter the number and kinds of drugs used and lower the price at which they are acquired from manufacturers and pharmacies. All of those tools, to

Box 2.

How a Medicare Drug Benefit Would Interact with Supplemental Drug Coverage

Roughly three out of four Medicare beneficiaries have drug coverage through such sources as employment-based health plans for retirees, state programs (including Medicaid), and individually purchased medigap policies. How those supplemental sources of coverage would operate after the introduction of a Medicare drug program would determine the extent to which the Medicare benefit stimulated demand for prescription drugs. It would also affect the ability of the benefit's administrators to use cost-management tools effectively.

Effect on People with Employment-Based Plans
Some beneficiaries who already have drug coverage through their employer could lose that coverage if a Medicare drug program was created. In recent years, employers have reduced the share of premiums they pay for retirees and, in some cases, have eliminated health benefits for retirees entirely. That trend could accelerate if a drug benefit was added to Medicare.

Employment-based drug coverage is typically more generous than the coverage envisioned under most of the recent proposals for Medicare. Thus, people who lost employment-based coverage might have an incentive to spend less on drugs under Medicare than they do now, because they would be paying more of the costs themselves.

Employers who kept a drug benefit for retirees would most likely provide it as a supplement to Medicare's coverage, as they already do for coverage of physician and hospital care. They would require beneficiaries to enroll in the Medicare drug program to retain their private coverage. The employment-based plan would probably reimburse beneficiaries for any difference between what it would have covered and what Medicare would cover. (For example, a plan that had no deductible might pay for beneficiaries' drug purchases below the deductible amount in Medicare.) Enrollees who continued to have access to generous supplemental coverage would have limited incentive to curb their drug spending under Medicare, regardless of the design of the benefit.

Effect on People in State Programs
Beneficiaries eligible for Medicaid or state-run pharmaceutical assistance programs would also have little reason to alter their spending on drugs. State Medicaid agencies would most likely enroll beneficiaries with dual eligibility in the Medicare drug program, since doing so would reduce the agencies' costs. (Those costs would decline because the premium for the Medicare drug benefit, which would be based on the average cost of all participants in the benefit, would probably be lower than the average cost of drugs for dual eligibles. If the federal government subsidized any of Medicare's drug premium, state Medicaid costs would decrease even more.) Like retiree health plans, Medicaid would supplement Medicare's drug coverage.

The Congressional Budget Office expects that state-based pharmaceutical assistance programs for low-income seniors would quickly be refocused once a Medicare drug benefit was in place. If the new Medicare benefit did not include premium and cost-sharing assistance for the programs' target groups, those programs might be redesigned to "wrap around" (supplement) Medicare, just as Medicaid would. Thus, a Medicare drug benefit would probably have little impact on those beneficiaries' demand for drugs, and the wraparound coverage could undermine any incentive to control costs that was built into the structure of the Medicare drug benefit.

Effect on People with Individual Drug Coverage
Only a small percentage of Medicare beneficiaries have private medigap policies that include drug insurance. As noted in Chapter 1, the drug coverage provided by those policies is expensive and limited, with annual benefits capped at either $1,250 or $3,000. Since medigap premiums are not subsidized and the plans have higher administrative costs than a Medicare plan probably would, medigap enrollees could get drug coverage through Medicare at lower cost. Thus, medigap plans with drug coverage as now structured would probably disappear, and new medigap plans (if allowed) would be developed to wrap around the Medicare drug benefit. Those wraparound provisions would stimulate demand for drugs and weaken the ability of Medicare to control costs. Conversely, prohibiting new medigap plans from offering drug coverage would help keep demand from rising.

one degree or another, work by influencing physicians' or consumers' choices about what drug to prescribe or where to fill a prescription.

Proposals that limit the scope of cost-management tools available to benefit managers would reduce the potential for controlling costs and demand. As an example of such limits, some recent proposals would require benefit managers to reimburse enrollees for a nonformulary drug if the prescribing physician certified that the drug was medically necessary. Other proposals would require that formularies include at least two drugs in each therapeutic class. Still others would limit the ability of benefit managers to exclude pharmacies from their network contracts.

Having a single PBM administer the Medicare drug benefit in each region, as some proposals envision, could pose problems for the use of formularies. If each PBM established its own formulary, enrollees in the Medicare drug program would have to pay different prices for the same drug solely on the basis of where they live. Those differences might not prove acceptable politically. Conversely, if Medicare adopted a nationwide formulary, that formulary would probably not be very restrictive, because nationwide exclusion from the Medicare market could threaten the profitability—and even the survival—of some drug manufacturers. (If the regions were large enough, exclusion of a drug from the formulary of even one region would also have significant financial implications for some manufacturers and might be difficult to sustain politically.)

Compromise approaches—such as limiting reimbursements for nonpreferred drugs only to the amount that would be paid for a therapeutically equivalent preferred drug—would probably make systems that steer patients toward certain drugs more acceptable under a single-PBM design. Such approaches could also save money if the cost-sharing requirements adopted under a proposal were flexible enough (see Appendix A).

An important limit on the ability of any benefit manager to control the costs of a Medicare drug benefit is the fact that some enrollees might continue to have extensive drug coverage through public programs or private health plans (see Box 2). If a supplemental insurer paid the bulk of an enrollee's drug copayment regardless of whether the drug was on the PBM's formulary or preferred-drug list, the usefulness of formularies and similar cost containment methods would diminish. The leverage that PBMs might have with pharmacies or manufacturers would be weakened as a result.

Insurance Risk and Competition

The incentive to control spending would be strong if the administering entity bore substantial insurance risk for delivering the benefit at or near some target cost. That situation would arise if the entity had to pay part or all of the extra cost when per-enrollee spending exceeded the target—and, conversely, got to keep at least part of the savings when that spending was less than the target. The incentive to curb costs would be even greater if the entities administering drug plans also had to compete with each other for enrollees on the basis of premiums and out-of-pocket drug costs. All other things being equal, enrollees would reward lower-cost plans with their business.

Although insurance risk and competition would encourage cost containment, they would also give plans more incentive to use management tools to achieve favorable selection than would be the case if a single plan was awarded a contract for all enrollees in a region. All plans would probably adopt similar tools as a defense against the use of such tactics by their competitors. However, there may be natural limits to the use of aggressive management tools by competing plans, because enrollees would choose among plans not only on the basis of premiums and costs but also on the basis of quality and service.

Some policymakers question the importance of competition and the assumption of insurance risk as ways to save money from managing a drug benefit. In the private sector, PBMs typically do not assume any insurance risk for the drug benefits they administer, but they are often given broad authority to use an array of management tools on behalf of a plan. They may also be subject to having a bonus added to—or a penalty subtracted from—their administrative fee according to how well they meet specific performance goals. A similar approach was envisioned in some of the recent proposals for a Medicare drug benefit, which called for a single PBM selected periodically to serve each region, with all of the insurance risk borne by Medicare.

Two important differences exist, however, between how employment-based health plans and the government might use a PBM to control costs. First, proposals for a Medicare drug benefit generally include statutory limits on the management tools that Medicare could require of PBMs. Employment-based plans, by contrast, can more easily change cost control strategies as circumstances dictate.

Second, and more important, the federal workers who would make decisions for the Medicare drug program face different incentives than private companies and their decisionmakers do. Most private employers who offer health coverage operate in a competitive marketplace, which requires them to keep costs down so they can price their products competitively while maintaining generous enough benefits to attract skilled workers. Medicare faces pressure to deliver promised benefits to enrollees; its incentives for cost containment are probably not as strong as those of a private employer.

Medicare drug proposals that call for multiple risk-bearing plans to compete for enrollees' business, with few restrictions on cost control mechanisms, have the greatest potential to constrain drug costs through management. However, the savings in drug costs would be partly offset by two kinds of additional costs: the cost of bearing insurance risk, and the marketing costs that competitive plans would have to incur. In the end, the degree to which those added expenses put a drag on cost management would depend on the details of the benefit design.

The Insurance-Risk Premium. A modest cost increase will occur whenever a drug program requires a private entity to bear insurance risk. In general, riskier enterprises need higher dollar returns to operate than less-risky ones do, because unless investors are compensated for bearing the extra risk, investment in those enterprises will dry up.[13] All private firms face risk in the normal course of

doing business (such as the risk of misjudging labor costs or the strength of competition). Those normal business risks are not likely to differ among proposals for a Medicare drug benefit. But a design that requires PBMs or other entities administering the benefit to bear insurance risk imposes a higher cost on such entities than does a design that leaves insurance risk in the hands of the government. That additional cost is referred to as the insurance-risk premium.

One source of insurance risk is uncertainty about such things as the increase in demand that would arise from better drug coverage or unexpected scientific advances that could boost drug spending. Another source of insurance risk is the possibility of adverse selection. If there was a single Medicare drug plan in each region, and if a large share of the eligible Medicare population enrolled in the drug program, that source of risk would be minimal. With multiple plans, however, the risk of adverse selection becomes a significant concern. As noted earlier, that concern would be greatest in the early years of the program, when plans would have little data from which to predict their enrollees' drug spending or the benefits offered by their competitors.

Assessing the size of the insurance-risk premium is difficult. On the one hand, growth in the use of new drugs can be hard to predict, and the possibility of ending up with enrollees who have above-average costs is worrisome.

On the other hand, traditional financial theory suggests that the premium should be small or even zero. The reason is that new Medicare drug plans would most likely become additional holdings in the diversified portfolios of large investors. Those diversified portfolios would be subject to financial risks for the economy as a whole but would be protected from the idiosyncratic risk of any particular investment. From the point of view of an investor holding such a portfolio, the firm-specific risks of Medicare drug plans would balance out the risks associated

---

13. One possible response to risk is to take actions to reduce it. For example, companies might take out insurance against uncertainties

in the market, or they might accumulate cash reserves to deal with contingencies. Such actions would directly increase the costs of doing business, which would mean higher prices, whereas a firm that declined those approaches would have to deliver higher returns to investors, which would also mean higher prices.

with other firms. Unless the insurance risks of the drug plans were correlated with the general financial risks of the economy, the risk premium for drug plans would be small.

In practice, however, insurance risk would probably give rise to real costs, which would be reflected in the premiums charged by competing plans. For instance, in an effort to avoid losses, managers might buy reinsurance, which is generally priced above its expected payouts in order to cover the reinsurers' own selection risks as well as their business costs. Managers might also try to accumulate reserves to cover possible losses. Although those reserves could be invested in interest-bearing assets, holding them would still entail costs.

In short, the risk premium would be an economic cost of any drug benefit that required a private entity to bear insurance risk. Uncertainty about trends in demand or technology would impose a cost on the entity that would require compensation. The risk premium would be higher for designs that envisioned competitive plans than for one in which a single plan bore insurance risk. Of course, the alternative—having the federal government bear insurance risk—would increase the government's uncertainty about its spending in any enrollment period and thus make budgeting for the Medicare drug program more difficult.

Plans' Marketing Costs. Competition would introduce additional expenses associated with marketing to and enrolling Medicare beneficiaries, which would not arise if a single plan administered the drug benefit in each area. In a competitive system, the government would inform beneficiaries that Medicare drug coverage was available to them. The competing plans would then have to provide specific information about their plans to beneficiaries. If plans were also responsible for enrolling beneficiaries and collecting their premiums, the cost of carrying out those administrative functions would be higher than under a single-plan system. Most single-plan designs would probably adopt the relatively seamless administrative process used for Part B of Medicare, in which beneficiaries are automatically enrolled unless they decline coverage, and uniform premium amounts are deducted from beneficiaries' monthly Social Security checks.

The extra administrative costs associated with competition could be reduced if plans were responsible for marketing but the government administered the enrollment and premium-collection processes. A uniform process would benefit from economies of scale. Moreover, the infrastructure for determining eligibility, enrolling people, and collecting premiums already exists in the Medicare program.

Effects on Drug Prices

Even with active cost management by plans, prices for some prescription drugs would rise as a result of a Medicare drug benefit. As noted above, insurance stimulates demand for covered drugs by reducing their cost to beneficiaries. If the pharmaceutical industry were perfectly competitive, manufacturers would probably respond to higher demand not by raising prices but by increasing production at little additional cost, at least in the long run. (Short-run shortages of supply might lead to higher prices, but competition would ensure that drug companies would invest in new production capacity to meet the higher demand.)

The pharmaceutical industry is far from perfectly competitive, however. Drugs are unique among health care products and services in that many are subject to unusually strong intellectual property rights, which protect their manufacturers from competition. Those rights stem not only from patents but also from the exclusive rights to sell drugs that the Food, Drug, and Cosmetics Act grants to drugmakers in certain situations. The Food and Drug Administration, whose primary responsibility is to ensure the safety and efficacy of drugs sold in the United States, also helps enforce those intellectual property protections. As long as a drug is protected from imitation by patent or other exclusive marketing rights, its manufacturer has a legal and well-enforced monopoly over the product.

In the case of many drugs, companies' monopoly power is limited because close substitutes for the drug are available. For example, among the widely used cholesterol-lowering agents known as statins, five different chemical entities, each protected by patents, have similar modes of action and effectiveness.[14] As a result, companies that sell those

---

14. Institute of Medicine, *Description and Analysis of the VA National Formulary* (Washington, D.C.: National Academy Press, 2000).

drugs often spend considerable sums to advertise and promote their products and must consider the competition in setting prices.

Occasionally, though, a specific drug offers unique clinical benefits of such magnitude that the only limit on its price is consumers' willingness or ability to pay.[15] Insurance effectively increases consumers' willingness or ability to pay for covered drugs, so a generous drug benefit—with low cost-sharing requirements, high benefit caps, or low catastrophic stop-loss limits—would make newly insured patients more tolerant of high prices. If a unique drug with major clinical benefits had a target population composed mainly of Medicare beneficiaries, a new benefit with a low catastrophic stop-loss limit could cause the drug's manufacturer to raise the current price or enter the market with a high launch price. (Medicare would have few ways to prevent very high prices for such drugs, apart from imposing direct price controls or threatening to deny or delay coverage. However, the threat of such constraints could increase uncertainty about the market for new drugs and thus discourage investment in pharmaceutical research and development.)[16]

Such exceptional cases aside, the most likely effect of a Medicare drug benefit would be only moderate price increases, and only for drugs with patent protection or exclusive marketing rights. One reason is that Medicare beneficiaries make up just part of the prescription drug market. A manufacturer who wanted to raise prices would have to weigh the higher revenue available from newly covered Medicare beneficiaries against the potential for lost market share among other buyers. A second reason is that since many Medicare patients have good drug coverage now, the effect on drug prices of even the most generous Medicare benefit would be diluted (because drug coverage is already reflected in current or expected prices).

Nevertheless, the potential for manufacturers of patent-protected drugs to raise prices underscores the importance of giving the entities charged with managing the benefit both the incentive and the authority to use cost-management tools. If PBMs or health plans could actively manage drug utilization through formularies or other strategies, they could closely scrutinize drugmakers' claims of clinical superiority. And by exploiting opportunities for price competition, they could hold pricing power in check when close substitutes existed.[17] Conversely, if PBMs or health plans were discouraged from actively managing the Medicare drug benefit in those ways, there would be fewer limits on price increases.

Administrative Feasibility

Most recent proposals for a stand-alone Medicare drug benefit envision having private entities administer the benefit, but they differ markedly in the functions that such entities would perform. Some proposals would require those administrators not only to play the roles that PBMs do in the private sector but also to compete for enrollees, bear insurance risk, and cope with federal (and possibly state) regulation of their activities. The willingness and ability of private entities to participate under those conditions would affect the speed with which a Medicare drug program could be implemented nationwide and its ultimate cost.

Plans' Participation in a Single-Plan, No-Risk Design

In a design (such as the Clinton Administration's plan) that envisions a single administrative entity for each part of the country, with the government bearing insurance risk, entities such as PBMs would compete for contracts to manage the drug benefit for everyone who enrolled in an area. The government would presumably issue a request for proposals for each region and award a contract to a single entity in that region using a bidding process. The bidding would determine how much the government

---

15. One drug with unique clinical benefits is alglucerase, which replaces an enzyme that is deficient in people who have Gaucher disease, a frequently disabling and sometimes fatal condition if not treated. A single company currently has the exclusive right to market alglucerase. For a description of the disease and therapies, see the Web site of Genzyme Therapeutics (www.genzyme therapeutics.com/cerezyme).

16. See Congressional Budget Office, *How Health Care Reform Affects Pharmaceutical Research and Development* (June 1994).

17. Even the first drug in a new therapeutic class can soon face competition from similar drugs or therapies. The introduction of a new class of pain relievers, known as Cox-2 inhibitors, is a case in point. The first molecule in the class was approved for marketing in the United States at the end of 1998. A second drug was approved only a few months later, in May 1999. Similar drugs are currently awaiting approval for marketing in the United States.

paid each entity for processing claims on a fee-for-service, no-risk basis.

The administrative functions required in a single-plan, no-risk design would be similar to the functions that PBMs now perform for employment-based health plans. Although certain features of that type of Medicare drug program could discourage some PBMs from bidding for contracts, it is likely that several large PBMs would be willing to participate. With the chance to manage drug claims for millions of Medicare beneficiaries at stake, PBMs would have an incentive to bid for contracts from the beginning, because the winning bidder in the initial competition would be awarded an exclusive, potentially multiyear contract and could thus have a competitive advantage in future bidding.[18] Managing the Medicare benefit might also give PBMs an advantage in competing for contracts with employment-based plans, because it would simplify the coordination of benefits for retirees.

Larger PBMs, with the infrastructure to administer broad pharmacy networks and negotiate with drugmakers for rebates, might have a competitive advantage over smaller PBMs. Thus, administration of the Medicare drug benefit might end up being concentrated among a few large PBMs. Such concentration would not necessarily lead to higher costs, since bigger PBMs might be able to achieve economies of scale that smaller ones could not. But unless enough potential bidders survived and the contracts were rebid periodically, the approach of having a single regional benefit manager could eventually reduce incentives for contractors to operate efficiently and for the government to continue to achieve savings through competitive contracting. The ultimate impact on Medicare costs is uncertain: it would depend largely on the dynamics of the competitive-bidding process used to award contracts.

Plans' Participation in a Competitive, Risk-Based Design
The question of participation is more complex in a design in which multiple entities would be competing for enrollees in a region and those entities bore the insurance

risk. Adopting risk-based payment would require PBMs to change their current business model to put more emphasis on cost control. (In the private sector, PBMs agree contractually to meet certain performance targets, such as specific price discounts and utilization rates, but they are not at risk for total spending. Employers or insurance companies have the responsibility for managing enrollment, bearing risks, and complying with state and federal regulations that govern health plans.) The need for greater emphasis on cost control under a risk-based approach would require some PBMs to restructure themselves and could delay or discourage their participation. For example, to compete as risk-bearing entities, most PBMs would probably need to develop partnerships with insurance companies and seek state licenses. Alternatively, PBMs could offer their traditional benefit-management services to insurance companies that would provide the Medicare drug coverage.

Another barrier to plans' participation in a competitive design would be uncertainty about adverse selection, particularly interplan adverse selection. Especially in the early years of the program, plans might be unable to gauge how much interplan-selection risk they would encounter or to know how effective their strategies to counter such risk would be. Managers might take a "wait and see" approach to participation. Even if plans modified their design to mitigate adverse selection, as described earlier, the number of competing plans might be fewer in the initial years.

Concerns About Regulatory Changes. Insurers have stated that they would be reluctant to offer Medicare drug plans out of concern that the federal government or state governments might modify the rules of enrollment after the fact.[19] In particular, they worry that over time, the Congress might allow exceptions to one-time enrollment because of pressure from constituents, thus undercutting the effectiveness of one-time enrollment in preventing adverse selection. Insurers have also expressed concern that state regulators might try to alter benefit packages or set other requirements that would impose unworkable limits on them.

---

18. See CBO's estimate of the Clinton Administration's prescription drug proposal in Congressional Budget Office, *CBO's Analysis of the Health Insurance Initiatives in the Mid-Session Review* (July 18, 2000).

19. See the testimony of Charles N. Kahn III, President, Health Insurance Association of America, before the House Committee on Ways and Means, June 13, 2000.

Actions by states to license and regulate drug plans could have a significant impact on plans' initial participation in the Medicare drug program. State insurance regulators might issue new rules for licensing such plans, including standards for financial solvency, that could vary widely from state to state. The time needed to obtain a license in each state would also vary. In addition, the relative speed with which states put requirements in place could affect start-up costs for plans trying to obtain licenses in multiple states. Moreover, depending on the type of prescription drug benefit enacted, state insurance regulations might affect the tools a plan could use to control drug costs, the procedures for enrollees to appeal decisions about coverage and to settle grievances, and the premiums that Medicare beneficiaries would pay for drug coverage. (For more information about current state laws that could affect Medicare drug plans, *see Box 3.*)

One way to work within those laws and possibly encourage the formation of nationwide plans would be to enact a federal preemption of state laws governing Medicare drug plans.[20] In addition, the federal administrator of the Medicare drug program could be given power to grant waivers of state insurance regulations. Waivers could be granted if states failed to process license applications quickly enough or if they imposed other barriers to licensing, such as requiring plans to meet more-stringent solvency standards than those established by federal regulation.

Participation by Medicare+Choice or Public Plans. One type of plan would be likely to participate from the beginning in a competitive, risk-based design: Medicare+Choice plans. Those plans have the marketing, enrollment, and customer-service infrastructure to compete for enrollees. They also have experience bearing insurance risk and working within the regulatory structure of the Medicare program. Providing drug coverage to Medicare beneficiaries could be done seamlessly through M+C plans as an enhancement of their basic benefits. In that case, however, drug coverage would be available only to

---

20. Alternatively, regulatory functions might be shared between the federal and state governments. For example, states might issue insurance licenses, and the federal government would regulate rates and benefits.

beneficiaries who enrolled in M+C plans for their basic Medicare benefits.

In some areas, it is possible that only one plan or even no plans would participate in the drug program. Without multiple plans in a region, the full benefits of competition would not be realized. If that happened, the government might have to provide its own public plan as a fallback in those areas to ensure a competitive benefit nationwide or, alternatively, provide additional financial incentives for private plans to operate in those regions. Fallback plans would be very vulnerable to interplan adverse selection in any region in which there was also a stand-alone drug plan or a Medicare+Choice plan. If the fallback plan was less aggressive than other plans in managing costs, the federal government could end up paying more, on average, in areas requiring such direct intervention.

Effects on Other Parts of Medicare

Adding a stand-alone prescription drug benefit to Medicare would have ripple effects on the rest of the program. With greater access to prescription drugs, some Medicare beneficiaries might use fewer health care services; in other cases, though, use of health care could increase. (The evidence that exists from past studies is inconclusive.) In all, costs for other Medicare services would probably not change significantly.

A drug benefit would also affect enrollment in Medicare's managed care plans (Medicare+Choice) by diluting one of their current competitive advantages—prescription drug coverage. However, M+C plans might be more likely to continue participating in Medicare because they would receive payment for their drug coverage rather than having to finance it themselves.

Impact on Other Medicare Services

By reducing financial barriers to the purchase of prescription drugs, a Medicare drug benefit would free up income for elderly people to use on other things, including additional health care. And by lowering the out-of-pocket price of prescription drugs for some enrollees, the benefit would stimulate demand for more, and possibly more costly, prescription drugs than before. Greater access to outpatient prescription drugs would improve the health

Box 3.

State Insurance Laws That Affect Prescription Drug Plans

A Medicare drug program that failed to preempt state insurance laws would subject participating plans to a wide array of regulations. Those regulations would make it more costly for plans to enter some markets, which could hinder the development of regional drug plans.

Many states have laws that would limit plans' ability to use certain tools—such as formularies and selective contracting with pharmacists—to control drug costs. As of December 2001, 26 states required health plans to have procedures whereby an enrollee can request coverage for drugs not on the plan's formulary. Eight states required plans, in certain cases, to continue covering drugs that are removed from the formulary.[1] In addition, 17 states had "any willing pharmacy" laws, which require managed care plans to contract with any pharmacy that is willing to meet the terms and conditions of the contract, and 16 states had "freedom of choice" laws, which prohibit plans from restricting enrollees' choice of pharmacies in return for a price discount. (Nine states had both types of laws.)[2] Plans administering the Medicare drug benefit in those states would face higher costs, which could result in higher premiums or cost-sharing amounts for enrollees.

Many states also regulate the procedures for enrollees in managed care plans to appeal decisions about coverage and to settle grievances. At the end of 2001, 41 states and the District of Columbia had laws mandating the establishment of an independent or external review process for consumers to appeal certain adverse judgments.[3] Laws in nine states allow an enrollee to hold a health plan accountable for its treatment decisions and to sue the plan in the appropriate civil court.[4]

Other state laws would affect the premiums that plans could charge for Medicare drug coverage. Ten states have enacted community-rating legislation, which requires health insurers to charge policyholders the same premium regardless of their health status or history of claims.[5] Twenty-nine states have laws that require plans selling health insurance in some markets to obtain prior approval of their rates from the state's insurance commission.[6]

---

1. Blue Cross Blue Shield Association, *State Legislative Health Care and Insurance Issues: 2001 Survey of Plans* (Washington, D.C.: BCBSA, 2001).

2. Health Policy Tracking Service, *2001 State by State Guide to Managed Care Law* (Washington, D.C.: National Conference of State Legislatures, 2001).

3. Henry J. Kaiser Family Foundation, *Assessing State External Review Programs and the Effects of Pending Federal Patients' Rights Legislation* (Menlo Park, Calif.: Kaiser Family Foundation, 2002).

4. Henry J. Kaiser Family Foundation, *Key Characteristics of State Managed Care Organization Liability Laws: Current Status and Experience* (Menlo Park, Calif.: Kaiser Family Foundation, 2001).

5. AARP Public Policy Institute, *Reforming the Health Care System: State Profiles 1998* (Washington, D.C.: AARP, 2000), and personal communication to the Congressional Budget Office by staff members of AARP, January 17, 2001.

6. National Association of Insurance Commissioners, *NAIC's Compendium of State Laws on Insurance Topics* (Kansas City, Mo.: NAIC, 2000), and personal communication to the Congressional Budget Office by staff members of the National Association of Insurance Commissioners, January 17, 2001.

of some seniors, which could reduce their use of hospitals and other services.

However, it is not clear that total costs for other Medicare services would decline. For one thing, greater use of drugs, especially in an older population, would increase the chances of side effects, allergic reactions, medication errors, and other adverse events—which could lead to new or longer visits to hospitals, emergency rooms, and other health care services.[21] To try to limit the frequency of adverse drug events for people on chronic therapies, physicians often require periodic visits and lab tests, and those precautions also raise costs.

A Medicare drug benefit could have a beneficial effect, however, on certain kinds of adverse drug events—those stemming from inappropriate dosing and interactions between drugs. Under most proposals, the benefit would be managed by entities that use electronic claims systems, which can identify and warn patients or prescribing physicians of potentially dangerous interactions when drugs are dispensed. That feature would be newly available not only to enrollees who now lack drug coverage but also to enrollees whose current coverage is not administered through such systems.

The evidence that is available to gauge how access to drug coverage affects health care costs is difficult to interpret. Few research studies address the question directly; rather, they examine the effects of a specific drug or class of drugs on health costs. Only a handful of studies have looked at the impact of drug coverage on health costs, and they have focused only on the most vulnerable and chronically ill subgroups of the population. Taken as a whole, the evidence from those studies is inconclusive.

Some recent research suggests that using more and newer drugs may reduce the use of other health care services; but other studies suggest that modest increases in financial access to drugs for elderly patients may not produce such a reduction. (For a more-detailed review of the research findings, see Appendix B.) New evidence may become available in the next year as researchers complete evaluations of state pharmaceutical assistance programs for the elderly.

Even if a drug benefit led to net savings in other Medicare costs, those savings would probably be relatively small, for two reasons. First, beneficiaries with Medicaid or employment-based insurance already have better coverage than would be available through many proposed Medicare drug benefits, so they would see little change in their drug use. And for their part, Medicare beneficiaries who lack drug coverage already use a significant quantity of prescription drugs. (On average, they filled 25 prescriptions in 1999, compared with 32 for Medicare beneficiaries who had drug coverage, CBO estimates.)[22] The additional, or more expensive, drugs that they might use as a result of gaining coverage would probably provide less-dramatic or less-immediate improvements in their health than do the drugs they are currently taking.

Second, any improvements in health would probably delay rather than prevent the use of expensive health care services. Delaying the onset of disability or end-of-life care is unquestionably a good thing, but it also means that what is saved in one year may be spent a few years later. Moreover, to the extent that a drug benefit helps people live longer, they may consume more health care over their remaining lifetime than they would have without the benefit.

---

21. See, for example, H. Kaisu and others, "Inappropriate Drug Prescribing in Home-Dwelling Elderly Patients," *Archives of Internal Medicine*, vol. 162 (August 12/26, 2002), pp. 1707-1712; R.R. Aparasu and S.E. Fliginger, "Inappropriate Medication Prescribing for the Elderly by Office-Based Physicians," *Annals of Pharmacotherapy*, vol. 31, no. 7-8 (July-August 1997), pp. 823-829; and General Accounting Office, *Adverse Drug Events: The Magnitude of Health Risk Is Uncertain Because of Limited Incidence Data*, GAO/HEHS-00-21 (January 2000).

---

22. That estimate is based on the 1999 Medicare Current Beneficiary Survey, with adjustments for underreporting and for use of drugs by beneficiaries in nursing homes and other long-term care facilities.

Impact on Medicare+Choice

As of August 2002, about 14 percent of Medicare beneficiaries were enrolled in Medicare+Choice plans.[23] In the past, those managed care plans were attractive to enrollees because they offered benefits beyond the basic Medicare package—the most desirable of which was prescription drug coverage. In recent years, however, changes in payment rates that have lagged behind growth in plans' costs have led some plans to withdraw from Medicare and others to raise enrollees' premiums or reduce drug coverage and other extra benefits. Consequently, enrollment in Medicare+Choice fell by 1.4 percent in 2001 after growing by 4.8 percent the previous year.

Adding a prescription drug benefit to Medicare would affect M+C plans in two ways. Plans that offer drug coverage would receive payment for the value of that coverage rather than having to finance it from their savings on administration or benefits. M+C plans have cited the rising cost of prescription drugs and the lack of Medicare payment for drug coverage—combined with the 1997 changes in payment rates—as reasons for dropping out of Medicare. Additional payment to cover the cost of a prescription drug benefit would help stabilize participation by M+C plans (in the absence of other disincentives to participate).

At the same time, the availability of drug coverage in regular fee-for-service Medicare would remove one of the principal incentives for new beneficiaries to select M+C plans. Such plans would have to differentiate themselves from fee-for-service Medicare through lower out-of-pocket costs, smaller premiums, or bigger benefits. However, the universal availability of drug coverage could give M+C plans a new competitive advantage over fee-for-service Medicare: because M+C plans provide the full package of Medicare benefits for enrollees, they would have greater flexibility than new plans that provided only drug benefits to substitute medical services for prescription drugs in a cost-effective manner.

23. Lori Achman and Marsha Gold, *Medicare+Choice and Medicare Beneficiaries: Monthly Tracking Report for August 2002*, no. 42 (Washington, D.C.: Mathematica Policy Research, September 5, 2002).

4

Cost Estimates for Specific Proposals

The various design choices described in Chapters 2 and 3 have a significant impact on the costs of a proposed Medicare drug benefit. The effects of those choices are complex and interdependent. To illustrate the overall impact, this chapter presents the Congressional Budget Office's cost estimates for four proposals, all of which were developed at the time of the 106th Congress (1999 to 2000). Those proposals are:

■ The drug benefit described in the Clinton Administration's June 2000 *Mid-Session Review;*

■ The Robb amendment (introduced by Senator Charles Robb as amendment 3598 to H.R. 4577);

■ H.R. 4680 (introduced by Congressman William Thomas), which passed the House of Representatives in October 2000; and

■ Breaux-Frist II (S. 2807, introduced by Senator John Breaux).

Those proposals cover a broad spectrum of approaches for delivering a Medicare drug benefit. For example, H.R. 4680 and Breaux-Frist II would have private-sector entities (such as pharmaceutical benefit management companies or health insurers) compete for enrollees and assume insurance risk for their drug spending. By contrast, the Clinton Administration's proposal would have those entities compete to be selected as the single nonrisk plan in each region to administer the Medicare drug benefit. Like H.R. 4680 and Breaux-Frist II, the Robb amendment

would have multiple plans compete for enrollees in each area, but they would not bear insurance risk.[1]

To estimate the costs of a proposed Medicare drug benefit, CBO uses a model that simulates how a given proposal would affect the spending of a representative sample of Medicare beneficiaries. The model contains detailed information about beneficiaries' spending for prescription drugs and Medicare-covered services, their supplemental insurance coverage (both public and private), their health status, and their income.[2] CBO's cost estimates result from the operation of that model; the effects of specific design choices cannot be quantified independent of a proposal's complete design specifications.

The primary factor that determines the federal costs of a given drug benefit is how much of enrollees' current drug spending the new Medicare benefit would cover. That amount, in turn, depends on the structure of the coverage and the number of people who would enroll. But CBO's

---

1. Under the Robb amendment, the Secretary of Health and Human Services could (but would not be required to) link a plan's payments to certain performance standards proposed by the plan in its bid to be allowed to offer the Medicare drug benefit. Those standards could include cost control. However, given the vagueness of the proposal's language, CBO has interpreted that provision as not requiring plans to bear insurance risk.

2. The estimates in this chapter are based on data from Medicare claims for 1999 and from the 1999 Medicare Current Beneficiary Survey, projected forward using CBO's March 2002 economic assumptions and baseline projections of Medicare spending.

estimates also assume that besides simply redistributing who pays for drug spending, the new benefit would cause enrollees to change their behavior. Some might fill more prescriptions or use more brand-name drugs once they gained better insurance coverage, thus increasing overall drug spending. The new Medicare benefit might also give manufacturers greater room to raise prices on certain drugs (if enrollees became less sensitive to the price of their prescriptions). Conversely, spending could fall if the entities that administered the drug benefit made aggressive use of cost-management tools, which can result in substantial price discounts and changes in the mix of drugs prescribed or purchased.

CBO's Key Assumptions

The issues discussed in the previous chapters would affect both the value of the drug benefit that enrollees receive and its costs to the federal government. CBO's approach takes those issues into account through six key assumptions that are incorporated in the estimating model:

■ *Beneficiary participation rate*—the percentage of Medicare beneficiaries who would enroll in the drug program. CBO assumes that the beneficiary participation rate is directly related to the share of total premium costs subsidized by the government.[3] The pool of potential enrollees includes beneficiaries who currently lack drug coverage, people who would use the new Medicare benefit to replace their private drug coverage, and those who would keep their private coverage as a supplement to the new Medicare benefit.

■ *Price effect*—the percentage increase in drug prices for the Medicare population that would gradually occur as a result of the new benefit. A benefit that covered a larger share of enrollees' total drug spending would tend to generate greater price increases than less comprehensive benefit packages would. (Any mitigating effect of cost management on price increases is captured in the cost-management factor described below.)

■ *Cost-management factor*—a measure of a proposal's potential for reducing spending on drugs below what would be spent by people whose purchases were not managed. The cost-management factor represents the net effect of an amalgam of price discounts and rebates, utilization controls, and other tools that a PBM might use to hold down spending. CBO assumes that PBMs would have greater incentive and ability to control spending under proposals in which they had to compete for enrollees and assume insurance risk for their spending and in which they had broad flexibility to manage enrollees' behavior through tools such as restrictive formularies.

■ *Induced demand*—the increase in enrollees' spending on prescription drugs as a result of the insurance coverage provided by the new Medicare benefit. CBO assumes that enrollees' drug spending would rise by 3 percent for each 10 percent drop in their out-of-pocket costs under the benefit.[4] As is the case with the price effect, induced demand is directly related to the relative generosity of the proposed drug coverage. The overall effect on spending per enrollee is the net result of induced demand, the price effect, and the cost-management factor.

■ *Marketing costs*—the additional costs associated with acquiring members and administering drug plans when multiple plans must compete for enrollees in each region. Those costs could be lower if plans used standardized marketing materials that allowed potential enrollees to compare plans more easily, with Medicare providing general information about the available choices. CBO assumes that marketing costs would be fairly high in the early years of a Medicare drug program because plans would need to make all Medicare beneficiaries in their area aware of their services. In later years, marketing costs would decline because plans would focus on smaller numbers of people (mainly those who were newly eligible for Medicare).

---

3. In CBO's model, "premium costs" refers to the total value of the benefits paid out plus the cost of administering the drug program.

4. In economists' terms, CBO assumes that the elasticity of demand for prescription drugs is -0.3. As used in this study, "out-of-pocket costs" include cost-sharing expenses but not an enrollee's share of premiums.

■ *Risk-premium costs*—a measure of the additional resources required by private plans if they bear insurance risk. Those resources could represent the pool of financial reserves needed to cover future drug claims if benefit spending is higher than a plan anticipates, or the price of private reinsurance that a plan would need in order to limit its risk, or both. CBO assumes that the risk premium would be higher in the initial years of a Medicare drug program because plans would have little data from which to predict the future cost of their benefits.

Details of Four Recent Proposals

This section looks at the key assumptions that CBO used for its cost estimates of four Medicare drug proposals introduced during the 106th Congress. For the past few years, when CBO has updated its 10-year projections of drug spending by or for Medicare beneficiaries, it has also updated its estimates for those proposals as a way to evaluate the results of its estimating models and reassess key assumptions. The four proposals are particularly useful for that effort because they represent a broad spectrum of approaches in terms of both the scope of the benefit packages and the diversity of ways in which Medicare might administer a drug program.

Because the four proposals were introduced several years ago, their original versions would have started the drug benefit in 2002 or 2003, giving Medicare two or three years to set up the program. For purposes of the estimates presented here, CBO assumes that each proposed benefit would begin in 2005.

In spite of the shift in timing, CBO retained the proposals' original values for deductibles, benefit caps, and limits on out-of-pocket spending, rather than adjusting them for inflation. For example, if a proposal called for a $250 deductible and a $5,000 stop-loss provision beginning in 2003, the estimates described here use those same values of $250 and $5,000 for 2005. (Each of the proposals calls for increasing the values of its benefit parameters after the first year of the program, which CBO also does in its estimates.) Keeping the same nominal values when drug spending is growing makes a proposal's deductible and stop-loss amounts relatively more generous, whereas keep-

ing the same value for a cap on benefits makes a proposal less so. As a result of that approach, most of the proposals examined here are more generous than when they were introduced.

All four proposals would offer the drug benefit as a voluntary program (called Part D of Medicare), but they would allow beneficiaries only a one-time opportunity to enroll without penalty. (If beneficiaries delayed enrollment, they would pay a penalty related to their expected benefit costs when they did sign up.) Without that provision, CBO would assume much lower rates of participation and much higher costs per enrollee for each proposal, because people would tend to postpone enrollment until their drug spending became relatively high.

In general, CBO assumes that all enrollees in Part B of Medicare would participate in a drug benefit that subsidized at least 50 percent of their premiums, so long as the proposed drug program met the following criteria:[5]

■ It offered a one-time option to enroll, coupled with an actuarially set penalty for late enrollment;

■ Beneficiaries were enrolled in the drug benefit by default;

■ Premium payments were withheld from an enrollee's Social Security check in the same manner that Part B premiums are withheld now;[6] and,

■ There were significant subsidies for low-income enrollees.

That approach includes a few exceptions, however. For example, CBO assumes that the 3 percent of Part B en-

---

5. CBO also assumes that Medicare beneficiaries who choose not to participate in Part B—where 75 percent of premiums are paid by the government—would refuse to enroll in any drug benefit with a lower subsidy rate.

6. CBO uses a higher subsidy "hurdle" when private plans rather than the Social Security Administration would administer the enrollment and premium-payment processes. In that case, a 75 percent federal subsidy would be necessary to achieve 100 percent participation.

Table 5.

Provisions of Four Prescription Drug Proposals for Medicare

	Clinton Mid-Session Review Plan	Robb Amendment	H.R. 4680	Breaux-Frist II
Benefit Amounts (Dollars)[a]				
Deductible	None	250	250	250
Benefit cap	1,000	None	1,050	1,050
Stop-loss amount	4,000	4,000	6,000	6,000
Benefit Administrator	SSA	SSA	Plans	SSA
Subsidies for Employment-Based Health Plans	Yes	Yes	No[b]	No[b]
Number of Plans in Each Region	One	At least two	At least two	At least two
Plans Bear Insurance Risk	No	No	Yes	Yes
Federal Subsidy for All Enrollees[c]	50% subsidy of premium costs below stop-loss amount; 100% above	50% subsidy of premium costs	No subsidy of premium costs; graduated reinsurance rate, averaging 35%[d]	25% subsidy of premium costs below stop-loss amount; 80% reinsurance above

Source: Congressional Budget Office.

Note: SSA = Social Security Administration.

a. The amounts that would apply in the Medicare drug benefit's first year of operation, which is assumed to be calendar year 2005.

b. Employment-based health plans for retirees could participate as entities that provide a Medicare drug plan, with the same federal subsidy as other plans. However, no attempt was made to estimate what share of total enrollment in the drug benefit they would account for.

c. "Premium costs" refers to the total value of the benefits paid out plus the cost of administering the drug program.

d. Today, the enrollee spending levels specified in H.R. 4680 at which federal reinsurance would be paid would lead to a federal subsidy of more than 35 percent. However, the legislative language caps that subsidy at 35 percent. Thus, the spending levels at which the federal government paid reinsurance would need to be raised.

rollees who are active workers and have drug coverage through their employer would keep that primary coverage rather than sign up for the Medicare benefit.[7] In addition, CBO assumes that Part B enrollees who also qualify for the Federal Employees Health Benefits (FEHB) program or the military's Tricare for Life (TFL) program would be less likely to participate in a new Medicare drug benefit because they already have fairly generous drug coverage. Unless FEHB and TFL beneficiaries were forced to enroll

---

7. That assumption is a simplifying one. Some of the 3 percent might enroll in a Medicare drug benefit, but under Medicare's secondary-payer rules, their employer's plan would pay first and thus would offset some of Medicare's costs.

in a Medicare drug plan (which current law would not permit), some might find that the premium for Part D was not worth the additional benefits.

The Clinton Administration's Proposal

The proposal included in the Clinton Administration's 2000 *Mid-Session Review* called for a Medicare drug benefit that would have no deductible and would pay 50 percent of an enrollee's drug spending up to a limit of $1,000 in 2005 (*see Table 5*). Once a participant incurred $4,000 in out-of-pocket costs during the year, Medicare would cover 100 percent of further drug spending. Under the proposal, plans would have the flexibility to vary their enrollees' coinsurance rates if they could demonstrate that the lower cost sharing would not raise costs for the Medicare program; that is, more-generous benefits would be offset by more-effective cost management.

The Secretary of Health and Human Services (HHS) would set a uniform national premium for the drug benefit. Under the Clinton proposal, enrollees' premiums would cover just half of a plan's benefit spending below the catastrophic cap and none of the spending above it. As a result, CBO estimates that if the drug program began operating in 2005, the federal government would subsidize 76 percent of benefit spending and administrative expenses for enrollees. Their share of premiums would amount to $30 a month in 2005, rising to $71 per month by 2012 (*see Table 6*).

Enrollees with income of up to 150 percent of the federal poverty level would receive assistance in paying their premiums; those with income of up to 135 percent of the poverty level would also get help in paying their cost-sharing amounts, including any spending above the benefit cap and below the stop-loss amount (the "hole"). In addition, Medicare would offer a subsidy to employment-based health plans to encourage them to remain the primary payer for their retirees' drug coverage. That subsidy would equal 67 percent of the premium subsidy that Medicare would have paid if a plan's retirees had enrolled in the Part D benefit.

CBO assumed that 86 percent of Part B enrollees would participate in the drug benefit, and another 7 percent would receive drug coverage indirectly through federal subsidies to employment-based plans. The remaining 7 percent of Medicare beneficiaries would not take part in the drug program but would continue to have drug coverage through their current employer, FEHB, or TFL.

Under the Clinton Administration's proposal, PBMs or other entities would compete to be the sole Medicare drug plan in each geographic area for a specified period of time. PBMs would not bear insurance risk for the drug spending of their enrollees, and they would face some restrictions in the cost containment approaches they could use. For example, they would have to set dispensing fees high enough to ensure participation by most retail pharmacies. In addition, enrollees would be guaranteed access to any drug that the prescribing physician certified as medically necessary. For those reasons, and because only one PBM would be chosen to serve each region, CBO assigned the proposal a relatively weak cost-management factor (10 percent).

CBO estimates that the Clinton Administration's plan would pay about 29 percent of the total drug costs of all Medicare beneficiaries—sufficiently generous to raise drug prices by about 8.5 percent above the level they would otherwise reach at the end of 10 years. In 2005, about 8 percent of Medicare's costs for the benefit would result from the greater use of drugs induced by the new coverage.

The Robb Amendment

Among the proposals examined here, the Robb amendment is the only one that would not cap an enrollee's benefits. Under that proposal, enrollees would pay a $250 deductible and graduated coinsurance rates—50 percent until their annual out-of-pocket spending for prescription drugs reached $3,500, then 25 percent until their out-of-pocket spending reached $4,000. After that amount, Medicare would cover 100 percent of any additional drug spending. The entities selected to administer the benefit would be allowed to waive the deductible for generic drugs and to lower enrollees' coinsurance rates if they could show that the lower cost sharing would be offset by effective cost management. The Robb plan also includes low-income subsidies to cover premiums and cost sharing for enrollees with income of up to 135 percent of the poverty level and premium assistance for people with income of up to 150 percent of the poverty level.

Like the Clinton Administration's plan, the Robb amendment would have the Secretary of HHS set a uniform nationwide premium. Federal subsidies would cover half of the cost of benefits and administrative expenses, with enrollees paying the other half through premiums. Their share of premiums would be about $67 per month in 2005, growing to $137 per month by 2012.

The Robb proposal would also offer to subsidize employment-based health plans if they remained the primary form of coverage for their retirees. Under that approach, Medicare would pay the plans 67 percent of the amount

Table 6.

CBO's Assumptions for Four Prescription Drug Proposals

	Clinton *Mid-Session Review* Plan	Robb Amend- ment	H.R. 4680	Breaux- Frist II
Values for Calendar Years 2005 Through 2012				
Percentage of Medicare Part B Enrollees Who Would Participate in the Drug Benefit				
Direct participation	86	85	75	87
Indirect participation (Through employer subsidy)	7	7	a	a
Percentage of Medicare Part B Enrollees Who Would Not Participate in the Drug Benefit				
People with other drug coverage[b]	7	7	7	5
People without other drug coverage	0	0	18	8
Total (All Medicare Part B Enrollees)	100	100	100	100
Cost-Management Factor[c] (Percent)	10	17.5	30	30
Federal Subsidy of Benefit Costs and Administrative Expenses for Enrollees in the Medicare Drug Program (Percent)	76	50	32	43
Share of Total Drug Spending by or for Medicare Beneficiaries Paid by the Federal Government (Percent)	29	21	12	15
Values for Calendar Year 2005				
Enrollees' Share of Monthly Premium (Dollars)	30	67	72	56
Plans' Marketing and Enrollment Costs (As a percentage of benefit spending)	0	7.8	13.5	11.9
Risk Premium[d] (As a percentage of benefit spending)	0	0	4.6	5.0
Percentage Increase in Drug Prices Expected Because of New Benefit[e]	0.9	1.5	*	0.1
Percentage of Benefit Costs Resulting from Increased Demand for Drugs Under New Benefit[f]	7.6	8.9	4.4	5.1
Values for Calendar Year 2012				
Enrollees' Share of Monthly Premium (Dollars)	71	137	119	95
Plans' Marketing and Enrollment Costs (As a percentage of benefit spending)	0	2.4	4.6	4.1
Risk Premium[d] (As a percentage of benefit spending)	0	0	3.3	3.6
Percentage Increase in Drug Prices Expected Because of New Benefit[e]	6.8	11.8	0.2	0.5
Percentage of Benefit Costs Resulting from Increased Demand for Drugs Under New Benefit[f]	9.6	8.7	3.9	4.7

Source: Congressional Budget Office.

Note: * = less than 0.05 percent.

a. Employment-based health plans for retirees could participate as entities that provide a Medicare drug plan, with the same federal subsidy as other plans. However, no attempt was made to estimate what share of total enrollment in the drug benefit they would account for.

b. Active workers with employment-based coverage or people covered by the Federal Employees Health Benefits program or the Tricare for Life program.

c. The percentage by which drug spending would fall relative to unmanaged purchases. For Breaux-Frist II and H.R. 4680, at-risk plans would have a cost-management factor of 30 percent, and fallback plans (5 percent or less of the total) would have a cost-management factor of 12.5 percent, for an average of about 29 percent. For people with supplemental drug coverage, the ultimate effect is a blend of Medicare's cost management and that of the supplemental plan.

d. The percentage of total benefit costs required to compensate plans for assuming insurance risk. CBO assumes that competing at-risk plans would require a risk premium equal to 7 percent of the benefits at risk in the first year of the program, declining to a steady state of 5 percent. Because of reinsurance provisions, 72 percent of benefits would be at risk under Breaux-Frist II, and 65 percent of benefits would be at risk under H.R. 4680.

e. The price effect is usually reported as the expected increase in prices at the end of a 10-year period. The 10th-year values for these proposals are 8.5 percent for the Clinton plan, 14.7 percent for the Robb amendment, 0.2 percent for H.R. 4680, and 0.6 percent for Breaux-Frist II.

f. For prescription drug spending, CBO assumes an elasticity of demand of -0.3, which means that enrollees' use of drugs is expected to increase by 3 percent for each 10 percent drop in out-of-pocket costs.

it would have paid in subsidies if the plans' retirees had enrolled in the new Part D drug benefit.

CBO assumed that 85 percent of Medicare Part B enrollees would participate in this proposal's drug benefit, and another 7 percent would receive coverage through the subsidy to employment-based plans for retirees. As under the Clinton proposal, the other 7 percent of Medicare beneficiaries would not participate in the drug benefit but would retain other coverage.

The Robb amendment envisions a competitive system, with at least two entities (selected through competitive bidding) administering the drug benefit in each region. Medicare would compensate PBMs by paying them an administrative fee. Those payments could be increased or decreased on the basis of whether the PBMs met certain performance standards, such as quality of service, enrollees' satisfaction, or targets for average spending per enrollee. PBMs could use restrictive formularies, subject to rules set by a national committee. However, all drugs approved for marketing in the United States would have to be provided if medically necessary, as established through procedures set by the PBM.

Under the proposal, at least two PBMs would compete for enrollees in each region, but they would not be subject to insurance risk for their enrollees' drug spending. Those plans would also have fewer explicit restrictions on the tools they could employ to control drug spending than under the Clinton Administration's plan. Consequently, CBO assigned the proposal a much higher cost management factor (17.5 percent) than the one for the Clinton plan.

Because of the structure of the proposed benefit, CBO assigned the Robb amendment the highest price effect of the four proposals—an increase of nearly 15 percent in drug prices by the end of 10 years. The Robb proposal would pay for about 21 percent of total drug spending by or for Medicare beneficiaries, CBO estimates. In 2005, about 9 percent of Medicare's costs for the benefit would come from enrollees' increased use of prescription drugs.

H.R. 4680

This proposal, which the House of Representatives passed in October 2000 but the Senate did not consider, also envisioned a drug benefit with a $250 deductible. Medicare would pay 50 percent of participants' drug costs, up to a cap of $1,050 in the first year of the benefit. Once enrollees incurred out-of-pocket costs of $6,000 or more during the year, Medicare would cover 100 percent of their drug spending. H.R. 4680 would allow participating plans to offer actuarially equivalent versions of the standard benefit—subject to certain limitations.

Low-income subsidies would cover premiums and cost-sharing expenses for enrollees with income of up to 135 percent of the poverty level, except that they would be responsible for covering any spending above the benefit cap and below the stop-loss amount. Enrollees with income of up to 150 percent of the poverty level would be eligible for assistance with their Part D premiums.

Once approved by the administering agency through a process of negotiation, plans would compete for enrollees in a region on the basis of premiums, access to drugs, and quality of service. Unlike the two proposals discussed above, H.R. 4680 would require those plans to assume significant insurance risk. It would also allow them to use a broad array of tools to control their enrollees' drug spending.

The federal government would ensure that at least two plans were available in each area, one of which could be a Medicare+Choice plan offering drug coverage. Employment-based health plans for retirees would also be eligible to participate directly as entities themselves. In any area not served by at least two plans, Medicare would have authority to offer financial incentives (such as a partial underwriting of risk) to encourage plans to operate in that region.

Rather than having one nationwide premium set by Medicare, H.R. 4680 would allow entities to set their own premiums. As a result, premiums would vary geographically and among plans. On average, enrollees would pay about $72 per month in premiums in 2005 and $119 per month by 2012.

Unlike in the other proposals, the federal government would not provide an across-the-board subsidy of each plan's premium. Instead, it would make reinsurance payments to plans for the spending of very high cost enrollees; in total, those payments would amount to 35 percent of the total cost of benefits paid out under the Part D program. Since plans would also incur costs for bearing risk and marketing to enrollees, CBO estimates that the federal government would pay for about 32 percent of plans' total spending.

Given that the proposal would offer a federal subsidy of less than 50 percent and that private entities would run the enrollment process and collect premium payments, CBO estimated that only about 75 percent of Part B enrollees would participate in the drug benefit under H.R. 4680. Another 7 percent of Part B enrollees would obtain drug coverage through their employer (because they are still active workers) or through FEHB or TFL. The remaining 18 percent of Medicare beneficiaries would not have drug coverage.

Compared with the other proposals, H.R. 4680 was assigned a relatively high cost-management factor (30 percent). The proposal would give plans greater incentive to control costs because they would be at risk for their enrollees' drug spending. They would also have relatively greater authority because they would face fewer restrictions on their cost-management tools. However, CBO estimates that a small share of enrollees (5 percent or less) would be served by fallback plans, which would bear much less risk and thus would not manage costs as tightly.

The benefit under H.R. 4680 would pay approximately 12 percent of Medicare beneficiaries' total drug costs. The relatively small benefit would cause very little increase in drug prices—0.2 percent by the end of 10 years, CBO estimates. Induced demand, which would result because certain enrollees gained better insurance coverage, would account for slightly more than 4 percent of Medicare's costs in 2005.

Breaux-Frist II
This proposal has the exact same benefit structure as H.R. 4680 and a similar subsidy for low-income enrollees, but

the federal subsidy for all enrollees differs. Whereas the House-passed bill would provide all of its federal subsidy through individual reinsurance payments for high-cost enrollees, Breaux-Frist II would subsidize 25 percent of premium costs below the $6,000 catastrophic cap and subsidize 80 percent of stop-loss benefits through individual reinsurance. CBO estimates that the combination of those two types of subsidies would total about 43 percent of premium costs.

Multiple risk-bearing plans would offer the benefit in each region, and premiums could vary geographically and among plans. (Enrollees' share of premiums would average $56 per month in 2005 and $95 per month in 2012, CBO estimates.)   However, unlike in H.R. 4680, the Social Security Administration would administer enrollment and collect premiums. Because of the higher federal subsidy and the near-automatic nature of SSA administration, CBO assumed higher participation: 87 percent of Part B enrollees. Another 5 percent would obtain drug coverage through their current employer, FEHB, or TFL, leaving 8 percent of Medicare beneficiaries without drug coverage.

PBMs would have the same incentives and authority to contain costs under this proposal that they would have under H.R. 4680, so CBO assigned the same cost-management factor (30 percent). Plans' marketing and enrollment costs would be somewhat lower under Breaux-Frist II than under H.R. 4680, because SSA would bear the cost of enrolling people and collecting their share of premiums. However, a plan's insurance-risk premium would cost more under this proposal because a higher share of total benefit costs would be at risk: 72 percent rather than 65 percent.

Although the two proposals envision identical benefit structures, Breaux-Frist II would have a slightly larger effect than H.R. 4680 would on drug prices (an increase of 0.6 percent by the end of a 10-year period) because of higher enrollment. In all, that proposal would pay for about 15 percent of total drug spending by or for Medicare beneficiaries. Induced demand for prescription drugs would account for about 5 percent of Medicare's costs in 2005.

Cost Estimates for the Four Proposals

Of the four proposals described above, the Clinton Administration's would be the most expensive, CBO estimates. It would cost the federal government a total of $512 billion between 2005 and 2012 (the last year of the current budget window), followed by the Robb amendment at $374 billion (*see Table 7*). The two proposals that have the same benefit structure but different federal subsidies, Breaux-Frist II and H.R. 4680, would be less costly to the federal government—$233 billion and $195 billion, respectively, over eight years. Those totals reflect additional costs for Medicare partly offset by savings for other federal programs.

The federal costs of a particular drug benefit depend largely on the extensiveness of the coverage and on what share of that coverage the government would pay for. Thus, the Robb and Clinton plans—which would pay for 20 percent to 30 percent of total drug spending by or for Medicare beneficiaries—would have the highest costs to Medicare. H.R. 4680 and Breaux-Frist II—which would pay 12 percent to 15 percent of Medicare beneficiaries' total drug costs—would have lower costs to the Medicare program.

A new Medicare drug benefit would affect not only Medicare's costs but also those of other federal programs—especially Medicaid, Tricare for Life, and the Federal Employees Health Benefits program. Any expansion of Medicare benefits would reduce those programs' health care costs for beneficiaries who were also eligible for Medicare. In the case of Medicaid, the federal government would have to pay less in matching contributions to state Medicaid programs for their spending on prescription drugs.

The savings to other federal programs from a Medicare drug benefit would be similar under the Clinton and Robb proposals—$145 billion and $142 billion, respectively, over the 2005-2012 period—because the two plans are nearly the same in terms of the scope of their drug coverage. Savings would be significantly smaller under H.R. 4680 and Breaux-Frist II—$84 billion and $78 billion, respectively—because those proposals would cover less of their enrollees' drug spending.

Each of the four proposals includes provisions that would subsidize all or part of the premium and cost-sharing expenses for low-income enrollees. As Table 7 shows, the

Table 7.
Federal Costs of Four Prescription Drug Proposals, 2005-2012

(By fiscal year, in billions of dollars)

	Clinton Mid-Session Review Plan	Robb Amendment	H.R. 4680	Breaux-Frist II
Federal Mandatory Spending on Prescription Drug Benefits for Medicare Beneficiaries				
Medicare	507	342	120	178
Other federal programs[a]	-145	-142	-84	-78
Low-income subsidy	128	148	141	123
Other Mandatory Spending	22	27	18	10
Total	**512**	**374**	**195**	**233**

Source: Congressional Budget Office.

Note: These numbers exclude a small amount of appropriated funds for federal administrative costs.

a. Principally Medicaid, the Federal Employees Health Benefits program, and the military's Tricare for Life program. Negative numbers indicate savings.

costs of those low-income subsidies can be quite large: in the case of H.R. 4680, surpassing even the costs to the Medicare program itself. The costs of the low-income subsidy are fairly similar among the four proposals—ranging from $123 billion to $148 billion over eight years. The reason for that similarity is that the differences in coverage among those Medicare drug benefits, which affect the subsidies for cost sharing, tend to be offset by differences in enrollees' premiums.[8] In other words, if a Medicare benefit covered less drug spending, the low-income subsidy would be responsible for picking up more enrollee cost sharing. However, premiums for such a benefit would also tend to be lower, offsetting some of the cost-sharing expense.

---

8. CBO's estimate for the Clinton proposal assumes that the low-income subsidy would pay all drug costs in the hole between the benefit cap and the catastrophic stop-loss limit. The Robb proposal has no such hole because it has no benefit cap. For H.R. 4680 and Breaux-Frist II, the low-income subsidies would not cover the hole.

In addition to the costs described above, a Medicare drug benefit would have other effects on federal spending. One is the additional cost that Medicaid and Medicare would incur if, as CBO expects, the low-income subsidies available under the drug benefit led more Medicare beneficiaries to apply for Medicaid benefits. Those new dual eligibles would increase costs for Medicaid, which would have to cover their cost-sharing expenses under Medicare. That increase would also raise Medicare's costs for those beneficiaries, because their use of covered services would rise. Another effect comes from provisions in certain proposals under which the federal government would keep some of the windfall savings that states would enjoy when a new Medicare drug benefit displaced state Medicaid drug spending. Such provisions tend to lower federal costs. A third effect is that of higher prices for prescription drugs in other federal programs (such as FEHB and TFL) that provide coverage to some Medicare enrollees. The line labeled "Other Mandatory Spending" in Table 7 shows the net impact of those effects.

A

Formulary-Based Strategies for Cost Control Used in the Private Sector

A key management tool that private-sector health plans and their pharmacy benefit managers (PBMs) use to control costs is drug formularies. A formulary is a list of drugs that a health plan will cover.[1] Formularies are generally created by pharmacy and therapeutics (P&T) committees that health plans (or employers that sponsor plans) establish to evaluate new drugs and to compare the clinical and economic characteristics of different drugs prescribed for the same medical condition. When a P&T committee judges two or more products to be therapeutically equivalent, it may recommend that only one of the products be included in the formulary. The health plan might pay part of its patients' costs for formulary drugs but would expect patients to pay the full price for any nonformulary drug—thus giving its enrollees a big incentive to choose formulary drugs. (Most plans that use a formulary have a process whereby enrollees can request exceptions to the formulary.)

Formularies can save money for health plans in two ways. First, to the extent that a formulary includes lower-priced drugs, any shift in prescribing patterns from nonformulary to formulary drugs will save money. Second, manufacturers may give price concessions—usually in the form of rebates—to a plan as an inducement to have their products included in the formulary.

---

1. Most hospitals also use formularies to determine what drugs they will stock or dispense. A formulary usually takes one of two forms: listing only those drugs that are covered (a closed formulary), or the mirror image, listing only those drugs that are not covered (an open formulary). This appendix focuses on closed formularies.

Drug-Preference Systems

In recent years, health plans have moved away from the traditional all-or-nothing formulary to a less rigid set of rules based on degrees of preference. In those preference systems, the health plan pays some share of the cost for all prescription drugs approved by the Food and Drug Administration (except any drugs specifically excluded, such as certain "lifestyle" drugs), but that share is larger for "preferred" drugs than for others. Preference systems still give enrollees an incentive to use preferred drugs, but the difference in out-of-pocket cost is not as great as with all-or-nothing formularies. Also, preference systems generally do not include a process for exceptions.

The way in which a plan computes its share of a drug's cost under a preference system is critical in determining how much the drug benefit will ultimately cost both the plan and its enrollees. Preference systems feature three basic reimbursement structures:

■ *Tiered copayments*, in which enrollees pay a fixed dollar copayment to a network pharmacy for drugs on the preferred list and a higher fixed copayment for other drugs (such as $10 per prescription for a preferred drug and $25 for a nonpreferred drug). For its part, the plan agrees to pay the pharmacy the difference between the full cost of the drug and that copayment. The full cost of the drug is usually negotiated with dispensing pharmacies in the PBM's network. Typically, that cost is based on an estimate of the pharmacy's cost of acquiring the drug's ingredients, plus a negotiated fee for dispensing the prescription.

- *Graduated coinsurance rates*, in which the plan pays the pharmacy a higher percentage of the full prescription cost for a preferred drug than for a nonpreferred drug (for example, 80 percent for a preferred drug and 50 percent for a nonpreferred drug). Enrollees pay the rest.

- *Reference pricing*, in which the plan pays the pharmacy a specified share of the full cost for a preferred drug and a dollar amount for a nonpreferred drug that equals what it would pay for a "reference" drug (a preferred drug that the P&T committee deems to be therapeutically equivalent to the nonpreferred drug). The enrollee pays the pharmacy the difference between the cost of the nonpreferred drug and the plan's share of the cost of the reference drug.

Tiered copayments are the arrangement used most frequently in private-sector drug plans today. In that system, the enrollee's financial exposure is capped at the highest copayment, and the enrollee's financial incentive to switch to a preferred drug is limited by the difference between the fixed copayments. The tiered-copayment system protects consumers against uncertainty about price differences between drugs when they enroll in a health plan and also against high out-of-pocket costs for very expensive drugs. However, it also partially shields consumers (or their physicians) from considering the trade-offs between medical benefits and price when wide differences exist between the actual prices of preferred and nonpreferred drugs.

Graduated coinsurance rates expose consumers to differences in drug prices more than tiered copayments do and thus make them more sensitive to price differences in their prescription choices. However, consumers are still insulated from the full price differences between preferred and nonpreferred drugs. Because enrollees' out-of-pocket costs vary with the price of a drug as well as with its status on the preferred list, enrollees can be uncertain about the extra cost associated with buying a nonpreferred drug.

Reference pricing exposes enrollees to the full price differences between preferred and nonpreferred drugs while still providing some reimbursement to enrollees who buy nonpreferred drugs. The greater the price difference be-

tween the preferred drug and its nonpreferred alternative, the more attractive the preferred drug appears. If the plan's contribution to the cost of the preferred drug is high, consumers will face little cost in obtaining that drug, even if it is very expensive. However, when they enroll in a plan, patients face uncertainty about how much they will have to pay for a nonpreferred drug, because that amount depends on the difference between its price and the price of the preferred drug. Plans, by contrast, have more certainty about their own spending than they do with either tiered copayments or graduated coinsurance rates, because their payment does not depend on the consumer's choice between preferred and nonpreferred drugs.

Effectiveness of Cost Control for Different Kinds of Drugs

A critical question is how effective each of those drug-preference systems would be in containing overall drug spending compared with an all-or-nothing formulary or with no formulary at all. Each system has certain advantages, which depend on the number and kinds of competing drugs in a therapeutic class.

Some drugs have little or no competition—not only because they are protected from generic copy by patents or other exclusive marketing rights but also because no similar drugs are available on the market. The first drug to treat a condition that hitherto had no available therapy would essentially be a one-of-a-kind member of a therapeutic class. As long as no close competitors were developed, neither formularies nor preference systems would have much effect on the price or use of that drug.[2]

Some therapeutic classes comprise several drugs, at least one of which has lost patent protection and is available in generic form. (Selective seratonin reuptake inhibitors,

---

2. Plans might resort to excluding certain new drugs from coverage. The threat of such exclusion could have much the same effect as formularies would on those drugs' initial prices. However, it would be politically difficult—as well as deleterious to patients' health—for the administrators of a Medicare drug benefit to exclude highly effective one-of-a-kind therapies on the basis of price alone.

which treat depression, are an example. Of the five distinct drug molecules in that class, two are available as generic copies.) When generic versions of at least one drug in a therapeutic class are available, reference pricing offers health plans the greatest opportunity to achieve cost savings in that class. Makers of generic drugs compete vigorously on the basis of the price at which they sell to pharmacies. If PBMs have good information about those prices, they can agree to pay network pharmacies a reference price at or near that level (adding an appropriate prescription-dispensing fee for the pharmacist). When enrollees choose to buy a brand-name version of a drug (or a competing drug that is not available in generic form), they must pay the full difference in price.

Some therapeutic classes contain only a few distinct drug molecules, all of which are protected by patents. (The new class of Cox-2 inhibitors, for example, contains only two drugs at present, Vioxx® and Celebrex®, although several other molecules have been submitted to the Food and Drug Administration for approval.) For small therapeutic classes such as those, reference pricing might not be as effective as tiered copayments in reducing costs. A tiered-copayment system lets a PBM require manufacturers of therapeutically equivalent drugs to bid for preferred status by offering rebates to the PBM. If the bidding is confidential, manufacturers will not know what their competitors may bid, so they will feel pressure to offer high rebates, and the PBM need not reveal the effective price offered by competing manufacturers.[3] With a reference-pricing system, by contrast, manufacturers of competing drugs would know (or soon learn) their competitors' prices. For therapeutic classes with only a few competitors, tacit price collusion could result, with all firms maintaining prices that were higher than they would have been under a tiered-copayment system.[4]

In the end, the amount that plans can save through different methods of enforcing formularies will depend on the copayments or coinsurance rates chosen for each tier, the number of tiers selected, and most important, the narrowness with which therapeutic classes are defined. If a P&T committee considers a broad array of drugs—of widely different ages and different mechanisms of action against the same disease—to be therapeutically equivalent, the opportunities for savings will be greater with reference pricing.

For example, if Cox-2 inhibitors were classified as part of the nonsteroidal anti-inflammatory class (which contains many old drugs with inexpensive generic versions available), a reference-pricing system in which a generic drug was preferred would cause the health plan to pay little for the Cox-2 drugs and consumers to bear a high share of the cost. Fewer enrollees would opt for Cox-2 inhibitors over the older, cheaper drugs. Conversely, if Cox-2 inhibitors were considered a distinct therapeutic class, the potential for savings would be lessened.

The trade-off for greater savings is that wide therapeutic classes containing drugs that have lost patent protection are more likely than narrow classes to reduce incentives for companies to invest in researching and developing new drugs.[5] If manufacturers believe that new drugs that make modest or even major clinical improvements will be classified in existing therapeutic classes, they will be discouraged from investing in such drugs by the prospect of lower returns. But at the other extreme, if classes are so narrowly defined that new drugs with small or even negligible improvements in effectiveness or safety are placed in their own separate class, drug companies will be encouraged to invest in new drugs that may not be cost-effective.

The effect of wide therapeutic classes on research and development would be greater under reference pricing than under tiered copayments. The reason is that a tiered-copayment system caps a patient's out-of-pocket payment, even for drugs that are not preferred, whereas refer-

---

3. That would probably not hold true with a Medicare drug benefit if Medicare required PBMs to pass on rebates to enrollees and the government at the point of each sale. Under such a rule, manufacturers would be able to learn what effective price the winning bidder had offered, so confidential bidding would be less successful in forcing price competition.

4. See F.M. Scherer, "How U.S. Antitrust Can Go Astray: The Brand Name Prescription Drug Litigation," *International Journal of the Economics of Business*, vol. 4, no. 3 (1997), pp. 239-256.

---

5. Patricia M. Danzon, "Pharmaceutical Benefit Management: An Alternative Approach," *Health Affairs*, vol. 19, no. 2 (March/April 2000), pp. 24-25.

ence pricing would place no upper limit on the patient's out-of-pocket cost. Thus, new drugs with high launch prices would have a greater disadvantage under a reference-pricing system with wide therapeutic classes than they would under a tiered-copayment system with the same therapeutic classifications.

B

Evidence About How Drug Coverage
Affects the Use of Other Health Care Services

A new Medicare drug benefit could lead to changes in the use—and, hence, the costs—of other health care services. People who argue that additional spending on prescription drugs would be at least partly offset by savings on other sources of health care (such as hospitals, physicians, and nursing homes) point to indirect evidence from three types of research:

- Studies of how specific drugs or classes of drugs affect the use of other health care,

- Studies of how improving access to prescription drugs (through insurance coverage) for vulnerable subgroups of the population changes their use of other health care services, and

- Studies of how the use of more or newer prescription drugs by defined populations affects their use of other health care services.

None of those approaches exactly address the question of how Medicare coverage for drugs might alter the use of other Medicare services. Moreover, the findings of those studies are conflicting and, in some cases, difficult to interpret.

Studies of Specific Drugs or Classes

Published studies of the impact of specific drugs or drug classes on the use of health care are, by definition, selective. Many of those studies have concluded that a partic-

ular drug or class of drugs would reduce, or has reduced, the use of expensive health care services.[1]

In general, such studies suffer from two methodological problems. First, they may be subject to publication bias—the tendency of authors to submit, and journals to publish, studies with findings that suggest improvements from therapy.[2] Second, many of those studies focus on groups of patients for whom the drug or drug class is approved for marketing (people who generally show the greatest positive effect from the drug) and exclude patient groups for whom the drug might be ineffective or even

---

1. See, for example, Samuel A. Bozzette and others, "Expenditures for the Care of HIV-Infected Patients in the Era of Highly Active Antiretroviral Therapy," *New England Journal of Medicine*, vol. 344, no. 11 (2001), pp. 817-823; and the Study of Left Ventricular Dysfunction (SOLVD) investigators, "Effect of Enalapril on Survival in Patients with Reduced Left Ventricular Ejection Fractions and Congestive Heart Failure," *New England Journal of Medicine*, vol. 325, no. 5 (1991), pp. 293-302.

2. See Mark Friedberg and others, "Evaluation of Conflict of Interest in Economic Analysis of New Drugs Used in Oncology," *Journal of the American Medical Association*, vol. 282, no. 15 (October 1999), pp. 1453-1457; and Carin Olson and others, "Publication Bias and Editorial Decisionmaking," *Journal of the American Medical Association*, vol. 287, no. 21 (June 5, 2002), pp. 2825-2828.

harmful.[3] Consequently, those studies provide little insight into the overall effect of changes in prescription drug coverage.

Studies of Changes in Access to Drugs

Only a handful of studies address the impact on health care use of a policy that alters access to prescription drugs. A major drawback of those studies is that they focus on the effects of reducing access to prescription drugs among subgroups of the population who have already been diagnosed with a chronic illness. A study that looked at the effects of increasing access to a wide variety of prescription drugs among a population that was more representative of all elderly people would be more useful in this case.

In 1981, New Hampshire changed its Medicaid rules by limiting to three the number of prescriptions that Medicaid patients could have filled in any month. A well-controlled study of that change found that the use of prescription drugs by elderly patients *who were on regular medication for chronic illnesses* declined as a result.[4] Their nursing home admissions increased, but their hospitalization rates did not. Because people in nursing homes were exempt from the three-prescription limit, the increase in nursing home admissions among chronically ill patients may have been an attempt to obtain needed drugs. The study did not examine all elderly patients who were subject to the limit; healthier individuals might have had fewer emergency and inpatient admissions because of reduced likelihood of harmful drug interactions, side effects, or other adverse drug events.

A more recent study of changes in a drug insurance program for the elderly focused on the Canadian province of Quebec, which restricted financial access to drugs by raising cost-sharing rates in 1996 and increasing deductibles in 1997.[5] That study found that use of prescription drugs declined in patients who, when the first policy change occurred, had been taking drugs deemed by a panel of clinicians to be "essential." Those patients also had an increased number of emergency room visits and admissions to hospitals or nursing homes. Patients taking drugs deemed "less essential" also saw their use of prescription drugs decline, but their use of other health care services did not increase. (Indeed, they showed a modest, but statistically insignificant, trend toward reduced hospitalization.) However, those two sets of drugs represented only about half of all prescriptions filled by the elderly; the effect of the restrictive financial policies on people taking other drugs was not studied. Thus, it is impossible from the study's results to assess the net effects of those restrictions on the use of other health care services among affected individuals.

Two studies of how state pharmaceutical assistance programs for low-income seniors affected the use of other health services found suggestive evidence that people enrolled in the programs used hospitals and other sources of health care less frequently than did other people studied.[6] However, because of data limitations, the methods used to control for competing factors that might account for those effects were crude. Consequently, the studies do not provide much insight into how a Medicare drug benefit could alter the use of other health care services.

---

3. Thomas Bodenheimer, *Conflict of Interest in Clinical Drug Trials: A Risk Factor for Scientific Misconduct* (Department of Health and Human Services, Office for Human Research Protections, August 15, 2000), available at http://ohrp.osophs.dhhs.gov/coi/bodenheimer.htm; and Laura F. Hutchins and others, "Underrepresentation of Patients 65 Years of Age or Older in Cancer-Treatment Trials," *New England Journal of Medicine*, vol. 341, no. 27 (December 30, 1999), pp. 2061-2067.

4. Stephen B. Soumerai and others, "Effects of Medicaid Drug-Payment Limits on Admission to Hospitals and Nursing Homes," *New England Journal of Medicine*, vol. 325 (October 1991), pp. 1072-1077.

5. Robyn Tamblyn and others, "Adverse Events Associated with Prescription Drug Cost-Sharing Among Poor and Elderly Persons," *Journal of the American Medical Association*, vol. 285, no. 4 (January 24/31, 2001), pp. 421-429.

6. Earle W. Lingle, K. Kirk, and W. Kelly, "The Impact of Outpatient Drug Benefits on the Use and Costs of Health Care Services for the Elderly," *Inquiry*, vol. 24 (Fall 1987), pp. 203-211; and Center for Health Policy Studies, *EPIC Evaluation Report to the Governor and Legislature: An Evaluation of New York State's Elderly Pharmaceutical Insurance Coverage Program* (Columbia, Md.: CHPS Consulting, no date).

Results were recently reported for a study that looked at the difference between three-tiered copayments and two-tiered copayments in the use of other medical services by enrollees in employment-based drug plans.[7] Moving from a two-tired to a three-tiered copayment system raises the cost of drugs not included on the preferred-drug list. The researchers found that in the year after the three-tiered system was introduced, drug use declined, but no significant differences in use of physicians, hospitals, or emergency medical services occurred. However, most of the enrollees were active workers and their dependents, who can be expected to be healthier and less dependent on prescription drugs than a Medicare population. Also, preferred drugs were determined by a pharmacy and therapeutics committee and presumably included only those classes of drug for which adequate choices exist.

Studies of the Effects of More and Newer Drugs

Two studies by Frank Lichtenberg provide suggestive evidence that increased use of prescription drugs and substitution of newer for older drugs are associated with lower use of hospitals and other health care services as well as lower mortality.[8] In particular, the second of those studies makes perhaps the strongest case that greater use of prescription drugs can lead to declines in nondrug health services. Yet even with Lichtenberg's relatively careful approach, that study's methodology may have underestimated each patient's nondrug health spending and thereby overstated the effects of newer drugs.

The first study related disease-specific changes in rates of hospital use between 1980 and 1991 to the change in the volume of prescriptions associated with each disease and to a disease-specific "drug novelty" index.[9] Increases in drug volume were correlated with reductions in hospital admissions, length of stay, and number of surgeries over the period. (The drug novelty index was also associated with declines in those measures of hospital use.)

One major problem with that study is that it assumed that unmeasured determinants of hospitalization rates—such as changes in hospital payment over the period—were not correlated with the degree of drug innovation (novelty) or with changes in drug use for a given diagnosis. But there is reason to believe that such correlation existed. Third-party payment and regulatory policies changed dramatically during the study period and encouraged reductions in days of hospital care.[10] Common diagnoses (such as cardiovascular disease) were likely to offer opportunities for big overall savings in hospital days as well as big markets for new drugs. Because the novelty index was based on switches among individual molecules, diseases with bigger markets would also be expected to have higher novelty indexes. Similarly, diseases with bigger markets might also provide greater financial incentives for the development of new diagnostic technologies, which would increase the number of people receiving therapy, and at earlier stages of the diseases. Thus, the study could be biased in favor of attributing too great a share of the decline in hospital utilization to increases in drug use and to the substitution of new drugs for old drugs.

The second study took a different tack. Lichtenberg hypothesized that people who took drugs that came on the market more recently would use less health care in 1996 (the year for which a survey of health care use was avail-

---

7. Brenda Motheral and Kathleen Fairman, "Effect of a Three-Tiered Prescription Copay on Pharmaceutical and Other Medical Utilization," *Medical Care*, vol. 39 (2001), pp. 1293-1304.

8. Frank R. Lichtenberg, "Do (More and Better) Drugs Keep People Out of Hospitals?" *Health Economics*, vol. 86, no. 2 (May 1996), pp. 384-388; and Frank R. Lichtenberg, *The Benefits and Costs of Newer Drugs: Evidence from the 1996 Medical Expenditure Panel Survey*, Working Paper No. 8147 (Cambridge, Mass.: National Bureau of Economic Research, 2001).

9. The drug novelty index was a measure of the change in the distribution of specific drug molecules prescribed between 1980 and 1991. An index value of zero meant no change in distribution between those years. A value of 1 meant no agreement at all in prescribing patterns between 1980 and 1991.

10. Most notably, in 1984, Medicare began using prospective payment for hospitals. It also required greater review of hospital admissions over the period. By 1991, the number of days of hospital care per 1,000 aged Medicare beneficiaries had declined to 2,672, from 3,846 in 1982; see "Medicare/Medicaid Statistical Supplement, 2000," *Health Care Financing Review* (June 2001), Table 23.

able) than would people who tended to take older drugs. Accounting for various characteristics of the patient and the condition for which a drug was prescribed, use of and expenditures for all other health care services were lower when newer drugs were prescribed than when older drugs were prescribed. The savings, especially in hospital costs, were substantially larger than the extra costs associated with using newer drugs.

The study did not account for hospital admissions or other health care that might have resulted from adverse drug events, because those admissions would often be for conditions not related to the purpose of the drug. (For example, an admission for liver failure resulting from long-term use of a cardiovascular drug would not be counted.) Thus, the study did not fully test whether cost savings from newer drugs outweighed cost burdens from adverse drug events. There are other technical questions about the methods used in the study. Nevertheless, the magnitude of the net savings estimated by Lichtenberg suggests that, on balance, patients who took newer drugs were likely to spend less on other kinds of medical care.